Gatford and Phillips'
Drug Calculations

Gatford and Phillips' Drug Calculations

Tenth edition

Julie-Anne Martyn
DipAppSci(Nurs), BNurs, MEd(T&D), PhD, SFHEA
Senior Lecturer in Nursing, School of Nursing, Midwifery and
Paramedicine, University of the Sunshine, Coast Fraser Coast,
Queensland, Australia

Matthew C. Carey
PhD, BSc, Dip-HE, PGCAP, fHEA, RCN
Lecturer in Nursing: Child Health, Faculty of Health: Medicine,
Dentistry and Human Sciences, School of Nursing and Midwifery,
University of Plymouth, Plymouth, United Kingdom

John D. Gatford
Mathematics Tutor, Melbourne, Australia

Nicole (Nikki) M. Phillips
DipAppSc(Nsg), BN, GDipAdvNsg(Educ), MNS, PhD
Professor of Nursing and Head of School, School of Nursing and
Midwifery, Deakin University, Victoria, Australia

ELSEVIER

Preface to the Tenth Edition

In this new edition, the structure of chapters has been revised to reflect the separation of medications into their forms and enhance reader knowledge of each concept. This begins with the introduction of a new Chapter 1: Forms of medication for calculation and administration. Revision has been made to chapters in the Ninth edition and re-titling of Chapters 3, 4 and 5. Sections from Chapters 3, 4 and 5 in the Ninth have been evaluated and aligned with each new chapter according to its relevant form of medication. Case scenarios have been added to Chapters 4 through to 6. The scenarios replace the revision sections at the end of each chapters in the Ninth Edition. The introduction of a new Chapter 7: Case scenario: the life of Maisy offers an across the lifespan case scenario for the patient Maisy to support theory into practice and consolidation to concepts explored in each chapter of the Tenth edition. This new chapter case scenario replaces the final revisions chapter from the Ninth edition. The revision of each chapter from the Ninth Edition has been reviewed and seen the removal and addition of questions throughout the text.

Matthew Carey and Julie Martyn
Queensland and England collaboration 2021

Preface to the First Edition

This book was written at the request of nurse educators and with considerable help from them. It deals with elements of the arithmetic of nursing, especially the arithmetic of basic pharmacology.

The book begins with a diagnostic test which is carefully related to a set of review exercises in basic arithmetic. Answers to the test are supplied at the back of the book, and are keyed to the corresponding review exercises.

Students should work through those exercises which correspond to errors in the diagnostic test. The other exercises may also, of course, be worked through to improve speed and accuracy.

Throughout the other chapters of the book there are adequate, well-graded exercises and problems. Each chapter includes several worked examples. Answers are given to all questions.

Suggestions and comments from nurse educators and students on the scope and content of this book would be welcomed. The hope is that its relevance to nursing needs will be maintained in subsequent editions.

J.D.G.
Melbourne 1982

Acknowledgements

We want to thank Elsevier for inviting us to contribute to this edition of the book we know is valuable for clinicians. We wish to acknowledge the validation from the user group and Elsevier for the changes made in this new edition.

We are grateful to the Sanofi—Aventis Group and to GlaxoSmithKline Australia Pty Ltd for permission to reproduce medication labels for inclusion in this book. Thank you to the Australian Commission on Safety and Quality in Health Care for granting permission to use the National Inpatient Medication Chart — Acute (2012).

Julie wants to thank Matt for collaboratively working for several months, across international timelines and with mutual respect and shared decision-making. We are a great team and now lifetime friends.

Matt wishes to thank Laura, Jacob and Evelyn for being themselves. He also wants to give special thanks to Julie for her guidance, support and friendship. We make a great team.

John Gatford wishes to thank his wife, Elaine, for her continuing support and patience during this ongoing project.

Thanks also, from Nicole Phillips, to Theo, Curtis, and Taylor.

Useful abbreviations

BSA	body surface area
cm	centimetre(s)
d.p.	decimal place(s)
g	gram(s)
hr(s)	hour(s)
hrly	hourly
IM	intramuscular
IV	intravenous
kg	kilogram(s)
kJ	kilojoule(s)
L	litre(s)
m^2	square metre(s)
mg	milligram(s)
mg/m^2	milligram(s) per square metre
mg/mL	milligrams per millilitre
mg/kg/day	milligrams per kilogram per day
min	minute(s)
mL	millilitre(s)
mL/hr	millilitres per hour
PCA	patient controlled analgesia
PO	orally
stat	immediately
subcut	subcutaneous
WFI	water-for-injection
%	percentage

Note: Do not use an abbreviation for micrograms.

Formulae used in this book

$$\text{Volume required (VR)} = \frac{\text{Strength required (SR)}}{\text{Stock strength (SS)}} \times \left[\begin{array}{c} \text{Volume of} \\ \text{stock solution (VS)} \end{array} \right]$$

$$\text{Volume (mL)} = \text{Rate (mL/hr)} \times \text{Time (hr)}$$

$$\text{Time (hr)} = \frac{\text{Volume (mL)}}{\text{Rate (mL/hr)}}$$

$$\text{Rate (mL/hr)} = \frac{\text{Volume (mL)}}{\text{Time (hr)}}$$

$$\text{Rate (mL/hr)} = \frac{\text{Volume (mL)} \times 60}{\text{Time (min)}}$$

$$\text{Rate (drops/min)} = \frac{\text{Volume (mL)} \times \text{Drop factor (drops/mL)}}{\text{Time (minutes)}}$$

$$\text{Rate (drops/min)} = \frac{\text{Volume (mL)} \times \text{Drop factor (drops/mL)}}{\text{Time (hours)} \times 60}$$

$$\text{Running time (hours)} = \frac{\text{Volume (mL)}}{\text{Rate (mL/hr)}}$$

$$\text{Concentration of stock (mg/mL)} = \frac{\text{Stock strength (mg)}}{\text{Volume of stock solution (mL)}}$$

$$\text{Dosage (mg)} = \text{Volume (mL)} \times \text{Concentration of stock (mg/mL)}$$

$$\text{Hourly dosage (mg/hr)} = \text{Rate (mL/hr)} \times \text{Concentration of stock (mg/mL)}$$

$$\text{Rate (mL/hr)} = \frac{\text{Hourly dosage (mg/hr)}}{\text{Concentration of stock (mg/mL)}}$$

$$\text{Weight of dextrose (g)} = \text{Volume of infusion (mL)} \times \text{strength of solution (g/100 mL)}$$

$$\text{Dose required (mg)} = \text{Body surface area (m}^2) \times \text{Recommended dosage (mg/m}^2)$$

Forms of medications for calculation and administration 1

CHAPTER CONTENTS

1. WHAT YOU NEED TO KNOW

In this chapter, you will learn about several forms of medication and the relationships between form, route and potency. You must know about the route of administration to understand how medications are absorbed, distributed, metabolized and excreted, also known as pharmacokinetics. The pharmacokinetics of a medication determines whether it acts locally or systemically. This knowledge is essential for the safety of administering medications by their different forms and routes. There are several administration routes that the prescriber can select. Usually, the route prescribed is considered the best for the patient's condition and capacity.

The routes of medication administration are as follows:

- *Enteral* means to give by the gastrointestinal tract. That could be orally or directly into the stomach by a feeding tube.
- The term *parenteral* means any route apart from the gastrointestinal tract. However, in contemporary practice, parenteral is understood to refer to 'by injection,' and could include intravenous, intramuscular, intradermal, or subcutaneous.
- *Topical* medications are transdermal, intravaginal, rectal, intranasal, transmucosal, sublingual, inhaled or administered into the eye or ear.
- *Neural* medications are administered as intrathecal, regional or epidural.

The potential for error is high with so many routes for medication administration. Therefore, when reading the prescription, pay attention to the route and think about whether it is appropriate for the patient under their current circumstances. For example, is the patient's swallowing reflex adequate to take solid oral medications safely? If not, you need to collaborate with the prescriber and discuss alternatives to a different forms and routes of medication? For example, the same drug may be in oral liquid form or suppository or as a liquid for parenteral injection.

2. FORMULATING MEDICATIONS

Formulating medications for administration by several routes is the role of a pharmacist. The prescriber can determine the form and route of the medication administration relevant to the patient. Finally, the person who administers the medication must confirm the accuracy and appropriateness of the prescription to treat the patient's condition.

In addition, and related to the calculation of medication dosages, having comprehensive knowledge of the form and route of medication for administration is essential for accurate dosage calculation. That is, the form and route of the medication will impact its potency. The therapeutic dosage is related to the medication form and route. Thus, you must understand the various forms of medication and how they are administered, to be able to determine correct calculation and measurement of the dosages. When medication prescriptions are changed the potency of the new form of medication must be known. Remember, an overdose can be dangerous, and too low a dose may result in a medication being ineffective. Attention to the prescribed form and route of medications is essential for safe practice.

Medications are available in solid, liquid, gel or gas forms.

3. SOLID MEDICATION FORMS

Solid medications are designed to deliver a single dose of medication and may come in these forms:

Tablet
Caplet
Capsule
Powder or granule

Lozenge
Pessary
Suppository

Tablets and capsules are clearly solid forms of medications. Powdered medications are solid as well, but they are prepared as small particles that sometimes can be atomized. For example, some inhaled medications are in powdered forms.

4. LIQUID MEDICATION FORMS

Liquid forms of medication are easier to identify. However, some liquid medications are for enteral administration and some are for parenteral. That is, some are taken orally, some are injected and yet others are drops for eyes and ears. Remember, you must know the intended route of administration because you must be able to differentiate the medication forms. For example, liquid antibiotics can be prepared as syrup for oral administration or a sterile liquid intended for intravenous administration.

Elixir
Syrup
Injectable sterile fluid

It would be disastrous to make a mistake and administer the oral form intravenously. Hence, you need to understand all aspects of medication forms, routes, potency and whether they are interchangeable. In many clinical settings, coloured syringes are used to differentiate their use for certain liquid medication administration forms. For example, oral syringes in the United Kingdom are coloured purple, whereas they can be orange or purple in Australia. In other circumstances, purple syringes are used for cytotoxic injectable medications. Thus, it is essential to familiarize yourself with these varying practices and abide by the local policy.

5. GEL MEDICATION FORMS

Gels can be classified as both solid and liquid forms, depending on their chemical composition. For example, the aloe vera plant produces a soothing gel that can be applied directly. Tea tree oil, on the other hand, requires modification and needs to be combined with other substances to produce a soothing gel. Gel medications are often water-based and semisolid. They are rapidly absorbed, depending on their form and route of administration. For example, a glycerin suppository will be absorbed faster than an ointment applied to the skin because of the available blood supply in the different body regions.

6. GAS MEDICATION FORMS

Medical gases are inhaled. They are absorbed and metabolized in the lungs. The alveolar circulatory system is extensive, and inhaled gases can enter the blood supply easily if the lungs are healthy.

⚠ *Important:* If in **any** doubt about the prescribed form of a medication, confirm the intention of the prescriber or a pharmacist.

Medications will act locally or systemically, depending on their form and route of administration. It is important for nurses to appraise the form of every medication critically *before* beginning to calculate the dose and prepare it for administration. That is, ask yourself, 'Is this the best way to give this patient this medication?'

7. ABSORPTION, DISTRIBUTION AND METABOLISM

To be able to calculate therapeutic medication dosages, you need to know about the body's absorption processes. Oral administration of medications is the most common and probably preferred method of taking medications. Most oral medications for adults are supplied as tablets or capsules; elixirs and syrups are most commonly used for paediatric patients. Solid medications must be broken down into smaller particles before they can be absorbed. That is, once swallowed, gastric acids in the stomach start to dissolve the solid form of the medication and the drug can be taken into the bloodstream by moving though the gastric mucosa to the liver drainage and into the circulatory system.

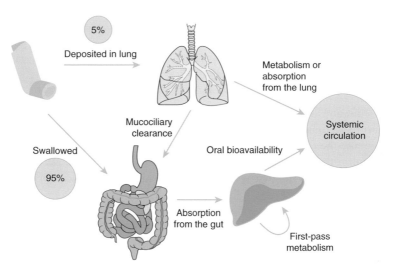

Figure 1.1 Absorption, distribution and metabolism pathway of a specific inhaled medication.

Example A

An explanation of the movement of medication follows using Fig. 1.1 as a diagrammatic representation of this example. An inhaled medication of 100 mg is administered. In this example, 95% (95 mg) of the medication is swallowed and is transported to the stomach. There, it is acted upon by enzymes to dissolve so that it can be absorbed through the gastric mucosa into the portal vein for distribution to the liver. The liver metabolizes the medication and deactivates 10% (9.5 mg) of the drug, leaving 85% (75.5 mg) of the unchanged drug available in the circulatory system.

Meanwhile, 5% (5 mg) of the medication was inhaled. The lungs metabolized 2.5% (2.5 mg) of the medication and transported the metabolite into the circulatory system through the alveolar membrane. The remaining 2.5% was swallowed after mucociliary clearance of the medication from the respiratory system. This 2.5% of the medication underwent hepatic first-pass metabolism in the liver, like the earlier 95% of the medication that was initially swallowed. The liver deactivated 10% of this secondary swallowed amount, leaving 2.25 mg of the active drug for processing and distribution to the circulatory system. Therefore, the bioavailability (that is, the amount that reached the bloodstream) was 75.5 mg (initially swallowed) + 2.5 mg (from the lungs) + 2.25 mg (secondarily swallowed) = 80.25 mg total active drug in the bloodstream for systemic circulation to the receptor cells in the body where it will act.

Note:

The bioavailability of medications will differ depending on how the medication is administered, as seen in Example A and Fig. 1.1. Therefore, oral dosages are often higher than intravenous dosages because of the process of first-pass metabolism. First-pass metabolism is the function of the liver to metabolize the medication in readiness for distribution by the blood stream to the receptor cells. Now, consider Example B (Fig. 1.2) in which an oral dose is different to that of the intravenous dose, but the bioavailability might be similar.

Example B

A 100-mg dose of oral morphine is given to patient A. It is swallowed whole and moves through the gastrointestinal tract, where it is dissolved and transported to the liver for metabolism. The liver produces active metabolites representing 80% of the original medication. These metabolites move to their respective receptors in the brain by the bloodstream. The time to reach an analgesic effect is about 20 min. Conversely, the same medication given by the intravenous route must be a much lower dose because of the potency of the medication is higher because it is injected directly into the bloodstream, and therefore bypasses the liver and the first pass metabolism process. That is, a 10-mg dose of morphine injected directly into the bloodstream will move quickly and act directly on brain receptors, with an immediate effect (Fig. 1.2).

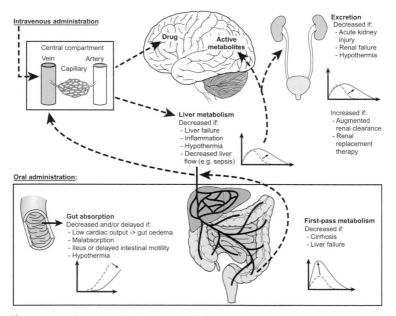

Figure 1.2 Absorption, distribution, metabolism and excretion pathway comparison of intravenous and orally administered medications.

Note in Fig. 1.2 that individual responses to medications will occur when there are physical factors that interfere with the function of the organs involved in administration, distribution, metabolism and excretion of medications.

8. MEDICATION ADMINISTRATION SAFETY

Understanding pharmacokinetics is an essential piece of knowledge to decipher the safety of medication dosage regimens. Remember that the form of a medication affects the therapeutic dosage required because of how the medication is administered, absorbed, distributed, metabolized and excreted by the body. The form to be administered depends on how the medication is prepared and supplied by a pharmacist, the patient's clinical need for the medication and the intention of the prescriber to treat the condition. You must understand all aspects of the medication to inform the decision-making process and accurately calculate and administer the medication safely.

Remember:

- Know the indication for the medication prescribed.
- Know the best route for the prescribed medication related to the clinical situation.
- Know the appropriate forms of the medication for the route that is prescribed.
- Ensure that the correct form is prescribed for the intended purpose.
- If there are concerns about the form of the prescribed medication, DO NOT administer it until you are clear about its indication.

2 | A review of relevant calculations

In this chapter, a list of mathematical terms is followed by a diagnostic test. This test is designed to pinpoint those areas of your arithmetic that need revising before you start nursing calculations. The test identifies what you already understand and what you need to review.

You should attempt all questions in the diagnostic test.

Answers are provided in Chapter 8. You will be directed to review exercises, depending on the incorrect answers in your diagnostic test.

For example, in the right-hand column in Chapter 8, you will see the specific exercises to review. If you make an error in answering either test question 1 or 2 on the diagnostic test, you will be directed to do Review exercise 2A. If your answer to test question 3 or 4 is wrong, you should do Review exercise 2B. You will not need to review any skills that the diagnostic test shows you already know.

Refer to prelim page ix for explanations of abbreviations.

1. MATHEMATICAL TERMS

WHOLE NUMBERS

Whole number: A number without fractions.

E.g., 5, 17, 438, 10, 592.

FRACTIONS

E.g., $\frac{3}{8}$, $\frac{17}{5}$, $\frac{1}{6}$, $\frac{9}{4000}$.

Numerator: The top number in a fraction.

E.g., in the fraction $\frac{3}{8}$, the numerator is 3.

Denominator: The bottom number in a fraction.

E.g., In the fraction $\frac{3}{8}$, the denominator is 8.

PROPER AND IMPROPER FRACTIONS

Proper fraction: A fraction in which the numerator is smaller than the denominator.

E.g., $\frac{1}{4}$, $\frac{5}{8}$, $\frac{11}{100}$.

Improper fraction: A fraction in which the numerator is larger than the denominator.

E.g., $\frac{5}{3}$, $\frac{32}{7}$, $\frac{100}{9}$.

An improper fraction can be converted to a mixed number.

E.g., $\frac{5}{3} = 1\frac{2}{3}$, $\frac{32}{7} = 4\frac{4}{7}$, $\frac{100}{9} = 11\frac{1}{9}$.

Mixed number: Partly a whole number, partly a fraction.

E.g., $1\frac{5}{8}$, $4\frac{1}{2}$, $10\frac{4}{5}$.

A mixed number can be converted to an improper fraction.

E.g., $1\frac{5}{8} = \frac{13}{8}$, $4\frac{1}{2} = \frac{9}{2}$, $10\frac{4}{5} = \frac{54}{5}$.

DECIMALS

Decimal: A number that includes a decimal point.

E.g., 6.35, 0.748, 0.002, 236.5.

Decimal places: Numbers to the right of the decimal point.

E.g., 6.35 has 2 decimal places.
     0.748 has 3 decimal places.
     0.002 has 3 decimal places.
     236.5 has 1 decimal place.

Place value: To the right of the decimal point are tenths, hundredths, thousandths, etc.

E.g., in the number 0.962, there are 9 tenths, 6 hundredths and 2 thousandths.

PERCENTAGES

Percentage: Number of parts per 100 parts.

E.g., 14% means 14 parts per 100 parts.
     2.5% means 2.5 parts per 100 parts.

A percentage may be less than 1%.

E.g., 0.3% = 0.3 parts per 100 = 3 parts per 1000.
     0.04% = 0.04 parts per 100 = 4 parts per 10,000.

OTHER TERMS

Divisor: The number by which you are dividing.

E.g., in the division 495 ÷ 15, the divisor is 15.

Factors: When a number is divided by another number and the answer is a whole number (i.e., there is no remainder), the divisor is a factor of the original number.

E.g.,   The factors of 12 are 1, 2, 3, 4, 6 and 12.
        The factors of 20 are 1, 2, 4, 5, 10 and 20.
        The number 1 is a factor of every number.

Common factors: Two different numbers may have common factors. A common factor is a divisor that is common to both numbers.

E.g., 1, 2 and 4 are the common factors of 12 and 20.

Simplify ('cancel down'): To write the number as *simply* as possible.

Calculate the value of: The answer will be a number.

2. DIAGNOSTIC TEST

Remember that this test is designed to help you meet your learning needs, so attempt the test questions without using a calculator. The online version of the text includes this diagnostic test with guidance to the answers after two attempts.

1. Multiply
   a. 83×10
   b. 83×100
   c. 83×1000

2. Multiply
   a. 0.0258×10
   b. 0.0258×100
   c. 0.0258×1000

3. Divide. Write answers as decimals.
   a. $3.78 \div 10$
   b. $3.78 \div 100$
   c. $3.78 \div 1000$

4. Divide. Write answers as decimals.
   a. $\dfrac{569}{10}$
   b. $\dfrac{569}{100}$
   c. $\dfrac{569}{100}$

5. Complete
   a. 1 kilogram = ... grams
   b. 1 gram = ... milligrams
   c. 1 milligram = ... micrograms
   d. 1 litre — .... millilitres

Be sure to include the unit of measurement in the answers to questions 6—11. Write the answers in decimal form where appropriate.

6. a. Change 0.83 kg to grams.
   b. Change 6400 g to kilograms.

7. a. Change 0.78 g to milligrams.
   b. Change 34 mg to grams.

8. a. Change 0.086 mg to micrograms.
   b. Change 294 micrograms to milligrams.

9. a. Change 2.4 L to millilitres.
   b. Change 965 mL to litres.

Check your answers in chapter 8.

10. a. Change 0.07 L to millilitres.

    b. Change 0.007 L to millilitres.

    c. Which is larger: 0.07 L or 0.007 litres?

11. a. Convert 0.045 g to milligrams.

    b. Convert 0.45 g to milligrams.

    c. Which is heavier: 0.045 g or 0.45 g?

12. Multiply
    a. 9×3 b. 0.9×3

    c. 0.9×0.3 d. 0.09×0.03

13. Multiply
    a. 78×6 b. 7.8×0.6

    c. 0.78×6 d. 7.8×0.06

14. Which of the numbers 2, 3, 4, 5, 6, 10, 12 are **factors** of 48?

15. Which of the numbers 2, 3, 5, 6, 7, 9, 11 are **factors** of 126?

16. Simplify ('cancel down')
    a. $\dfrac{16}{24}$ b. $\dfrac{56}{72}$ c. $\dfrac{45}{600}$

    d. $\dfrac{175}{400}$ e. $\dfrac{60}{90}$ f. $\dfrac{1600}{4000}$

17. Simplify ('cancel down'). Leave answers as improper fractions:
    a. $\dfrac{65}{20}$ b. $\dfrac{275}{50}$ c. $\dfrac{500}{80}$

    d. $\dfrac{700}{120}$ e. $\dfrac{400}{125}$ f. $\dfrac{600}{250}$

18. Simplify. Leave answers as improper fractions, where these occur:
    a. $\dfrac{0.6}{0.9}$ b. $\dfrac{0.45}{0.5}$ c. $\dfrac{200}{4.5}$

    d. $\dfrac{0.09}{0.05}$ e. $\dfrac{37}{0.4}$ f. $\dfrac{1.5}{15}$

Check your answers in chapter 8.

19. Round off each number correct to one decimal place:
    a. 0.68   b. 1.82   c. 0.35

20. Write each number correct to two decimal places:
    a. 0.374   b. 2.625   c. 0.516

21. Change to exact decimal equivalents:
    a. $\dfrac{5}{8}$ b. $\dfrac{9}{20}$

    c. $\dfrac{17}{25}$ d. $\dfrac{31}{40}$

22. Change to decimals correct to one decimal place:
    a. $\dfrac{1}{6}$ b. $\dfrac{3}{7}$ c. $\dfrac{7}{9}$

23. Change to decimals correct to two decimal places:
    a. $\dfrac{5}{7}$ b. $\dfrac{5}{9}$

24. Divide. Calculate the value of each fraction to the nearest whole number:
    a. $\dfrac{95}{3}$ b. $\dfrac{225}{4}$

25. Divide. Calculate the value of each fraction correct to one decimal place:
    a. $\dfrac{55}{6}$ b. $\dfrac{65}{9}$

26. Change to mixed numbers:
    a. $\dfrac{17}{2}$ b. $\dfrac{67}{3}$ c. $\dfrac{113}{5}$

27. Change to improper fractions:
    a. $2\dfrac{3}{4}$ b. $12\dfrac{5}{6}$ c. $28\dfrac{2}{5}$

28. Multiply. Simplify where possible:
    a. $\dfrac{2}{3} \times \dfrac{5}{6}$ b. $\dfrac{5}{8} \times \dfrac{12}{7}$ c. $\dfrac{9}{10} \times \dfrac{4}{9}$

Check your answers in chapter 8.

29. Multiply. Simplify where possible. Write each answer as a fraction, a mixed number or a whole number:

    a. $\dfrac{5}{4} \times 3$ b. $\dfrac{5}{8} \times 4$

30. Multiply. Give each answer as a decimal number:

    a. $\dfrac{11}{20} \times 4$ b. $\dfrac{30}{50} \times 2$

31. Convert to 24-hour time:
    a. 10:30 a.m.   b. 9:15 p.m.

32. Convert to a.m./p.m. time:
    a. 0730 hrs   b. 1850 hrs

33. What is the time 10 hrs after 2145 hrs on a Saturday?

Check your answers in chapter 8.

3. MULTIPLICATION BY 10, 100 AND 1000

To multiply whole or decimal numbers by 10, move the decimal point 1 place to the right.

To multiply whole or decimal numbers by 100, move the decimal point 2 places to the right.

To multiply whole or decimal numbers by 1000, move the decimal point 3 places to the right.

 Example

a. 0.36×10

b. 0.36×100

c. 0.36×1000

a. $0.36 \times 10 \quad = \overset{\frown}{3.6} \quad = 3.6$

b. $0.36 \times 100 \quad = \overset{\frown}{36.} \quad = 36.$

c. $0.36 \times 1000 = \overset{\frown}{360.} \quad = 360.$

Notes:

* Use zeros to make up places, where necessary. See the working of example c.
* If the answer is a whole number, the decimal point may be omitted. See the answer in example b.

 Memorize

To multiply by	Move the decimal point
10	1 place right
100	2 places right
1000	3 places right

✏ Review exercise 2A *Multiply*.

1. 0.68 × 10
   0.68 × 100
   0.68 × 1000

2. 0.975 × 10
   0.975 × 100
   0.975 × 1000

3. 5.62 × 10
   5.62 × 100
   5.62 × 1000

4. 77 × 10
   77 × 100
   77 × 1000

5. 825 × 10
   825 × 100
   825 × 1000

6. 0.2 × 10
   0.2 × 100
   0.2 × 1000

7. 0.046 × 10
   0.046 × 100
   0.046 × 1000

8. 0.0147 × 10
   0.0147 × 100
   0.0147 × 1000

9. 0.006 × 10
   0.006 × 100
   0.006 × 1000

10. 0.075 × 10
    0.075 × 100
    0.075 × 1000

11. 0.08 × 10
    0.08 × 100
    0.08 × 1000

12. 0.0505 × 10
    0.0505 × 100
    0.0505 × 1000

Check your answers in chapter 8.

4. DIVISION BY 10, 100 AND 1000

To divide whole or decimal numbers by 10, move the decimal point 1 place to the left.

To divide whole or decimal numbers by 100, move the decimal point 2 places to the left.

To divide whole or decimal numbers by 1000, move the decimal point 3 places to the left.

Example A

a. **37.8 ÷ 10**	a. $37.8 \div 10 = 3.\overset{\frown}{7}8 = 3.78$
b. **37.8 ÷ 100**	b. $37.8 \div 100 = 0.\overset{\frown}{3}78 = 0.378$
c. **37.8 ÷ 1000**	c. $37.8 \div 1000 = 0.\overset{\frown}{0}378 = 0.0378$

 Notes:

- To complete the division process, use zeros to make up places where necessary, as in example c.
- For numbers less than one, write a zero before the decimal point.

🧠 Memorize

To divide by	Move the decimal point
10	1 place left
100	2 places left
1000	3 places left

Example B

Division arithmetic may be written as a fraction in which the numerator is divided by the denominator.

a. $\dfrac{0.984}{10}$

b. $\dfrac{0.984}{100}$

c. $\dfrac{0.984}{1000}$

a. $\dfrac{0.984}{10} = 0.0984$

b. $\dfrac{0.984}{100} = 0.00984$

c. $\dfrac{0.984}{1000} = 0.000984$

Review exercise 2B *Divide. Write answers as decimals*

---

1. $98.4 \div 10$
   $98.4 \div 100$
   $98.4 \div 1000$

2. $5.91 \div 10$
   $5.91 \div 100$
   $5.91 \div 1000$

3. $2.6 \div 10$
   $2.6 \div 100$
   $2.6 \div 1000$

4. $307 \div 10$
   $307 \div 100$
   $307 \div 1000$

5. $82 \div 10$
   $82 \div 100$
   $82 \div 1000$

6. $7 \div 10$
   $7 \div 100$
   $7 \div 1000$

7. $\dfrac{68}{10}$
   $\dfrac{68}{100}$
   $\dfrac{68}{1000}$

8. $\dfrac{2.29}{10}$
   $\dfrac{2.29}{100}$
   $\dfrac{2.29}{1000}$

9. $\dfrac{51.4}{10}$
   $\dfrac{51.4}{100}$
   $\dfrac{51.4}{1000}$

10. $\dfrac{916}{10}$
    $\dfrac{916}{100}$
    $\dfrac{916}{1000}$

11. $\dfrac{89.4}{10}$
    $\dfrac{89.4}{100}$
    $\dfrac{89.4}{1000}$

12. $\dfrac{0.707}{10}$
    $\dfrac{0.707}{100}$
    $\dfrac{0.707}{1000}$

Check your answers in chapter 8.

5. CONVERTING UNITS

Metric units of mass, weight and volume are commonly used in
nursing calculations. You must memorize their conversions.

 Memorize

---

1 kilograms (kg) = 1000 grams (g)
1 gram (g) = 1000 milligrams (mg)
1 milligram (mg) = 1000 micrograms*
1 litre (L) = 1000 millilitres (mL)

Note: Always write micrograms in full to avoid
misinterpretation errors.

Example A *Kilograms to grams*

Change 0.6 kg to grams.

$$0.6 \text{ kg} = 0.6 \times 1000 \text{ g}$$
$$= 600 \text{ g}$$

Example C *Grams to milligrams*

Change 0.67 g to milligrams.

$$0.67 \text{ g} = 0.67 \times 1000 \text{ mg}$$
$$= 670 \text{ mg}$$

Example B *Grams to kilograms*

Change 375 g to kilograms.

$$375 \text{ g} = 375 \div 1000 \text{ kg}$$
$$= 0.375 \text{ kg}$$

Example D *Milligrams to grams*

Change 23 mg to grams.

$$23 \text{ mg} = 23 \div 1000 \text{ g}$$
$$= 0.023 \text{ g}$$

Example E *Milligrams to micrograms*

Change 0.075 mg to micrograms.

0.075 mg = 0.075 × 1000 micrograms

= 75 micrograms

Example F *Micrograms to milligrams*

Change 185 micrograms to milligrams.

185 micrograms = 185 ÷ 1000 mg

= 0.185 mg

Example G *Litres to millilitres*

Change 1.3 L to millilitres.

1.3 L = 1.3 × 1000 mL

= 1300 mL

Example H *Millilitres to litres*

Change 850 mL to litres.

850 mL = 850 ÷ 1000 L

= 0.85 L

⚠️ **Health professionals must be competent converters of units of measure to ensure accurate dosage calculations, because medications, fluids and dietary supplements are supplied in several forms and strengths.**

🖊 **Review exercise 2C** *Change (convert). Write all answers in decimal form.*

Change to grams:
1. 5 kg   2. 2.4 kg   3. 0.75 kg   4. 1.625 kg

Change to kilograms:
5. 7000 g   6. 935 g   7. 85 g   8. 3 g

Change to milligrams:
9. 4 g   10. 8.7 g   11. 0.69 g   12. 0.02 g
13. 0.006 g   14. 0.655 g   15. 4.28 g

Change to grams:
16. 7250 mg   17. 865 mg   18. 2 mg

Change to micrograms:
19. 0.6 mg   20. 0.75 mg   21. 0.075 mg   22. 0.08 mg
23. 0.001 mg   24. 0.625 mg

Change to milligrams:
25. 825 micrograms   26. 65 micrograms
27. 10 micrograms   28. 5 micrograms
29. 200 micrograms

Change to millilitres:
30. 2 L   31. 30 L   32. $1\frac{1}{2}$ L   33. $4\frac{1}{2}$ L
34. 1.6 L   35. 2.24 L   36. 0.8 L   37. 0.75 L

Change to litres:
38. 4000 mL   39. 10,000 mL
40. 625 mL   41. 95 mL
42. 5 mL

Check your answers in chapter 8.

6. COMPARING MEASUREMENTS

Example A

1 L = 1000 mL

Question
a. Change 0.4 L to milliliters.
b. Change 0.04 L to milliliters.
c. Which is larger: 0.4 L or 0.04 L?

Answer
a. 0.4 L = 0.4 × 1000 mL = 400 mL
b. 0.04 L = 0.04 × 1000 mL = 40 mL
c. 0.4 L is larger than 0.04 L

Example B

1 kg = 1000 g

Question
a. Convert 4.3 kg to grams.
b. Convert 4.03 kg to grams.
c. Which is heavier: 4.3 kg or 4.03 kg?

Answer
a. 4.3 kg = 4.3 × 1000 g = 4300 g
b. 4.03 kg = 4.03 × 1000 g = 4030 g
c. 4.3 kg is heavier than 4.03 kg

✎ Review exercise 2D *Change and compare*

Change each measurement in columns a and b to the smaller unit specified in the next questions. Then, decide which of those measurement is largest and write it in column c. See chapter 8 for the correct answers.

Change each measurement in columns a and b to millilitres (mL); then, choose the larger volume (c).

	a.	b.	c.
1.	0.1 L	0.01 L	
2.	0.003 L	0.3 L	
3.	0.05 L	0.005 L	
4.	0.047 L	0.47 L	

Convert each measurement in columns a and b to milligrams (mg); then, choose the larger weight (c).

	a.	b.	c.
5.	0.4 g	0.004 g	
6.	0.06 g	0.6 g	
7.	0.07 g	0.007 g	
8.	0.63 g	0.063 g	

Rewrite each measurement in micrograms; then, choose the larger weight (c).

	a.	b.	c.
9.	0.002 mg	0.02 mg	
10.	0.9 mg	0.09 mg	
11.	0.001 mg	0.1 mg	
12.	0.58 mg	0.058 mg	

Change each measurement to grams (g); then choose the heavier weight (c).

	a.	b.	c.
13.	1.5 kg	1.05 kg	
14.	2.08 kg	2.8 kg	
15.	0.95 kg	0.095 kg	
16.	3.35 kg	3.5 kg	

Check your answers in chapter 8.

7. MULTIPLICATION OF DECIMALS

Note: d.p. stands for decimal place(s).

Example A

a. 8×4
b. 0.8×4
c. 0.8×0.4

d. 0.08×0.04

a. $8 \times 4 = 32$
b. $37.8 \div 1000 = 0.0378 = 0.0378$
c. $0.8 \times 0.4 = 0.32$

$$1 \text{ d.p.} + 1 \text{ d.p.} \Rightarrow 2 \text{ d.p.}$$

d. $0.08 \times 0.04 = 0.0032$

$$2 \text{ d.p.} + 2 \text{ d.p.} \Rightarrow 4 \text{ d.p.}$$

Example B

a. 67×4
b. 6.7×0.4

c. 0.67×4

d. 6.7×0.04

a. $67 \times 4 = 268$
b. $6.7 \times 0.4 = 2.68$

$$1 \text{ d.p.} + 1 \text{ d.p.} \Rightarrow 2 \text{ d.p.}$$

c. $0.67 \times 4 = 2.68$

$$2 \text{ d.p.} + 0 \text{ d.p.} \Rightarrow 2 \text{ d.p.}$$

d. $6.7 \times 0.04 = 0.268$

$$1 \text{ d.p.} + 2 \text{ d.p.} \Rightarrow 3 \text{ d.p.}$$

Example C

a. **16 × 12**
b. **1.6 × 1.2**
c. **0.16 × 0.12**
d. **0.016 × 1.2**

a. $16 \times 12 = 192$
b. $1.6 \times 1.2 = 1.92$ (2 d.p.)
c. $0.16 \times 0.12 = 0.0192$ (4 d.p.)
d. $0.016 \times 1.2 = 0.0192$ (4 d.p.)

Review exercise 2E *Multiply*

1. 9×5
   0.9×5
   0.9×0.5
   9×0.05

2. 2×7
   0.2×0.7
   0.2×0.07
   0.02×0.07

3. 3×4
   3×0.04
   0.3×0.4
   0.03×0.04

4. 7×8
   0.7×8
   0.7×0.8
   0.07×0.08

5. 17×6
   1.7×6
   0.17×6
   0.17×0.6

6. 19×8
   19×0.8
   0.19×0.8
   1.9×0.08

7. 29×5
   0.29×5
   2.9×0.5
   29×0.05

8. 31×3
   3.1×0.3
   0.31×0.03
   31×0.003

9. 37×9
   3.7×9
   3.7×0.09
   0.37×0.09

10. 41×7
    0.41×0.7
    0.41×0.07
    4.1×0.7

11. 56×11
    5.6×1.1
    0.56×0.11
    56×0.011

12. 64×12
    6.4×0.12
    0.64×0.12
    0.064×1.2

Check your answers in chapter 8.

8. FACTORS

Many calculations involve simplifying (or 'cancelling down') fractions.

Simplifying fractions requires knowledge of *factors*. When a number is divided by one of its factors, the answer is always a whole number (i.e., there is no remainder).

 Note: The symbol ∴ means 'therefore'.

Example

Which of the numbers 2, 3, 5, 7, 11 are factors of 154?

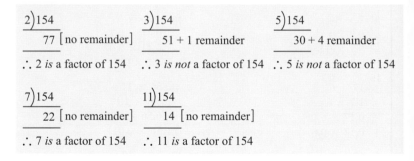

2, 7 and 11 are factors of 154.

 Note: These are not the *only* factors of 154.

Review exercise 2F *Which of the numbers in column B are factors of the opposite number in column A?*

	A	**B**
1.	20	2, 3, 4, 5, 7, 8
2.	36	3, 4, 5, 10, 12, 16
3.	45	3, 5, 7, 11, 12, 15
4.	56	2, 5, 8, 11, 14, 16
5.	60	3, 4, 8, 12, 15, 20
6.	72	3, 4, 6, 12, 15, 18
7.	75	3, 5, 7, 11, 15, 25
8.	85	3, 5, 9, 11, 15, 17
9.	96	3, 8, 12, 14, 16, 24
10.	100	3, 5, 8, 20, 25, 40
11.	108	4, 7, 9, 12, 16, 18
12.	120	3, 5, 9, 12, 15, 16
13.	135	3, 5, 7, 9, 11, 15
14.	144	4, 8, 12, 16, 18, 24
15.	150	4, 5, 9, 12, 15, 25

Check your answers in chapter 8.

9. SIMPLIFYING FRACTIONS I

To simplify (or 'cancel down') a fraction, divide the numerator *and* denominator by the *same* number. This number is called a *common factor*.

Nurses need to know how and when to simplify fractions because some medication dosage calculations use formulas that include fractions. For example, to calculate an intravenous infusion rate for a pump, the hourly rate of millilitres of liquid to be infused is found by dividing the volume to be infused by the time (in hours) of the infusion. It is shown as Rate = Volume/Time.

Notes:

- The *numerator* is the top number in a fraction.
- The *denominator* is the bottom number in a fraction.
- A *common factor* is a divisor that is common to more than one number.

Example A

Simplify $\dfrac{36}{48}$

$$\frac{36}{48} = \frac{3}{4} \quad \left[\begin{array}{l}\text{dividing numerator and} \\ \text{denominator by 12}\end{array}\right]$$

Or the same fraction may be simplified in several steps:

$$\frac{36}{48} = \frac{18}{24} \quad \left[\begin{array}{l}\text{after dividing numerator and} \\ \text{denominator by 2}\end{array}\right]$$

$$= \frac{9}{12} \quad \left[\begin{array}{l}\text{after again dividing numerator and} \\ \text{denominator by 2}\end{array}\right]$$

$$= \frac{3}{4} \quad \left[\begin{array}{l}\text{after dividing numerator and} \\ \text{denominator by 3}\end{array}\right]$$

Note: $2 \times 2 \times 3 = 12$ example in the second method. The sum of the steps noted here is equal to the denominator used in the previous example.

Example B

Simplify $\dfrac{125}{225}$

$$\frac{125}{225} = \frac{25}{45} \quad \left[\begin{array}{l} \text{after dividing numerator and} \\ \text{denominator by 5} \end{array} \right]$$

$$= \frac{5}{9} \quad \left[\begin{array}{l} \text{after again dividing numerator and} \\ \text{denominator by 5} \end{array} \right]$$

Gatford and Phillips' Drug Calculations

Review exercise 2G *Simplify ('cancel down')*

Part i *Simplify*

1. $\dfrac{8}{2}$

2. $\dfrac{10}{14}$

3. $\dfrac{6}{16}$

4. $\dfrac{9}{18}$

5. $\dfrac{15}{21}$

6. $\dfrac{20}{24}$

7. $\dfrac{20}{25}$

8. $\dfrac{12}{28}$

9. $\dfrac{28}{32}$

10. $\dfrac{22}{33}$

11. $\dfrac{14}{42}$

12. $\dfrac{42}{48}$

13. $\dfrac{36}{56}$

14. $\dfrac{52}{64}$

15. $\dfrac{21}{70}$

Part ii *Simplify*

1. $\dfrac{75}{150}$

2. $\dfrac{75}{200}$

3. $\dfrac{75}{250}$

4. $\dfrac{125}{250}$

5. $\dfrac{125}{300}$

6. $\dfrac{125}{400}$

7. $\dfrac{30}{225}$

8. $\dfrac{40}{175}$

9. $\dfrac{60}{375}$

10. $\dfrac{375}{500}$

11. $\dfrac{275}{400}$

12. $\dfrac{100}{225}$

13. $\dfrac{175}{225}$

14. $\dfrac{225}{300}$

15. $\dfrac{425}{600}$

16. $\dfrac{375}{750}$

Check your answers in chapter 8.

10. SIMPLIFYING FRACTIONS II

When the common factor is 10 and the numerator and denominator both end in zero, you can simplify the fraction first by removing the zero from the numerator and denominator, which effectively divides both numbers by their common factor, which is 10 (see Example A).

Example A

Simplify $\dfrac{900}{1500}$

$$\dfrac{900}{1500} = \dfrac{9}{15} \quad \left[\begin{array}{l}\text{after dividing numerator and} \\ \text{denominator by 100}\end{array}\right]$$

$$= \dfrac{3}{5} \quad \left[\begin{array}{l}\text{after dividing numerator and} \\ \text{denominator by 3}\end{array}\right]$$

Example B

Simplify $\dfrac{1400}{4000}$

$$\dfrac{1400}{4000} = \dfrac{14}{40} \quad \left[\begin{array}{l}\text{after dividing numerator and} \\ \text{denominator by 100}\end{array}\right]$$

$$= \dfrac{7}{20} \quad \left[\begin{array}{l}\text{after dividing numerator and} \\ \text{denominator by 2}\end{array}\right]$$

Review exercise 2H *Simplify ('cancel down')*

*Divide the numerator **and** denominator by 10 or 100 or 1000 (whichever is appropriate). Then, simplify further if possible:*

1. $\dfrac{30}{50}$

2. $\dfrac{40}{60}$

3. $\dfrac{50}{120}$

4. $\dfrac{100}{120}$

5. $\dfrac{130}{150}$

6. $\dfrac{60}{150}$

7. $\dfrac{120}{160}$

8. $\dfrac{60}{160}$

9. $\dfrac{200}{300}$

10. $\dfrac{270}{300}$

11. $\dfrac{450}{500}$

12. $\dfrac{120}{500}$

13. $\dfrac{1400}{2500}$

14. $\dfrac{1750}{2500}$

15. $\dfrac{2500}{3000}$

16. $\dfrac{500}{3000}$

17. $\dfrac{1200}{4000}$

18. $\dfrac{2750}{4000}$

Check your answers in chapter 8.

11. SIMPLIFYING FRACTIONS III

Leave answers as *improper fractions*.

Example A

Simplify $\dfrac{175}{50}$

$$\frac{175}{50} = \frac{35}{10} \quad \left[\begin{array}{l} \text{after dividing numerator and} \\ \text{denominator by 5} \end{array}\right]$$

$$= \frac{7}{2} \quad \left[\begin{array}{l} \text{after again dividing numerator and} \\ \text{denominator by 5} \end{array}\right]$$

Example B

Simplify $\dfrac{400}{120}$

$$\frac{400}{120} = \frac{40}{12} \quad \left[\begin{array}{l} \text{after dividing numerator and} \\ \text{denominator by 10} \end{array}\right]$$

$$= \frac{10}{3} \quad \left[\begin{array}{l} \text{after dividing numerator and} \\ \text{denominator by 4} \end{array}\right]$$

Review exercise 21 *Simplify ('cancel down')*

Leave answers as improper fractions.

1. a. $\dfrac{30}{20}$ b. $\dfrac{50}{20}$ c. $\dfrac{75}{20}$ d. $\dfrac{85}{20}$

2. a. $\dfrac{100}{8}$ b. $\dfrac{150}{8}$ c. $\dfrac{300}{8}$ d. $\dfrac{750}{8}$

3. a. $\dfrac{150}{12}$ b. $\dfrac{350}{12}$ c. $\dfrac{500}{12}$ d. $\dfrac{1000}{12}$

4. a. $\dfrac{100}{40}$ b. $\dfrac{300}{40}$ c. $\dfrac{380}{40}$ d. $\dfrac{550}{40}$

5. a. $\dfrac{70}{50}$ b. $\dfrac{75}{50}$ c. $\dfrac{120}{50}$ d. $\dfrac{125}{50}$

6. a. $\dfrac{80}{60}$ b. $\dfrac{150}{60}$ c. $\dfrac{750}{60}$ d. $\dfrac{1000}{60}$

7. a. $\dfrac{100}{80}$ b. $\dfrac{200}{80}$ c. $\dfrac{550}{80}$ d. $\dfrac{1000}{80}$

8. a. $\dfrac{180}{120}$ b. $\dfrac{200}{120}$ c. $\dfrac{300}{120}$ d. $\dfrac{450}{120}$

9. a. $\dfrac{200}{125}$ b. $\dfrac{300}{125}$ c. $\dfrac{800}{125}$ d. $\dfrac{900}{125}$

10. a. $\dfrac{150}{125}$ b. $\dfrac{350}{125}$ c. $\dfrac{550}{125}$ d. $\dfrac{950}{125}$

11. a. $\dfrac{180}{150}$ b. $\dfrac{225}{150}$ c. $\dfrac{400}{150}$ d. $\dfrac{950}{150}$

12. a. $\dfrac{800}{250}$ b. $\dfrac{900}{250}$ c. $\dfrac{1200}{250}$ d. $\dfrac{1800}{250}$

Check your answers in chapter 8.

12. SIMPLIFYING FRACTIONS IV

To simplify a fraction involving decimals, multiply the fraction by $\frac{10}{10}$ or $\frac{100}{100}$, depending on the number of decimal places needed to make a whole number. If the number of decimal places is *higher* than (or *equal to*) one decimal place, multiply by $\frac{10}{10}$ (see Example A). If two decimal places are evident, multiply by $\frac{100}{100}$ (see Example B). Example C has no decimal places in the numerator and 1 decimal place in the denominator, so multiplying by $\frac{10}{10}$ to move the denominator decimal place will achieve a whole number and enable simplification of the fracture.

Note: d.p. stands for decimal place(s).

Example A

Simplify $\dfrac{0.4}{0.6}$

$\dfrac{0.4}{0.6} \begin{array}{l} \leftarrow 1 \text{ d.p.} \\ \leftarrow 1 \text{ d.p.} \end{array}$ $\left[\begin{array}{l} \text{both numerator and} \\ \text{denominator have 1 d.p.} \end{array}\right]$

$\dfrac{0.4}{0.6} \times \dfrac{10}{10} = \dfrac{4}{6} = \dfrac{2}{3}$

Example B

Simplify $\dfrac{0.35}{0.4}$

$\dfrac{0.35}{0.4} \begin{array}{l} \leftarrow 2 \text{ d.p.} \\ \leftarrow 1 \text{ d.p.} \end{array}$ $\left[\begin{array}{l} \text{numerator has 2 d.p.;} \\ \text{denominator has 1 d.p.} \end{array}\right]$

$\dfrac{0.35}{0.4} \times \dfrac{100}{100} = \dfrac{35}{40} = \dfrac{7}{8}$

Example C

Simplify $\dfrac{100}{2.5}$

$\dfrac{100}{2.5}$ ← 0 d.p.
← 1 d.p. $\left[\begin{array}{l}\text{numerator has 0 d.p.;}\\ \text{denominator has 1 d.p.}\end{array}\right]$

$\dfrac{100}{2.5} \times \dfrac{10}{10} = \dfrac{1000}{25} = \dfrac{200}{5} = \dfrac{40}{1} = 40$

Example D

Simplify $\dfrac{0.07}{0.02}$

$\dfrac{0.07}{0.02}$ ← 2 d.p.
← 2 d.p. $\left[\begin{array}{l}\text{both numerator and}\\ \text{denominator have 2 d.p.}\end{array}\right]$

$\dfrac{0.07}{0.02} \times \dfrac{100}{100} = \dfrac{7}{2}$ $\left[\begin{array}{l}\text{leave answer as}\\ \text{an improper fraction}\end{array}\right]$

Review exercise 2J *Simplify. Answers may be left as improper fractions, where these occur. However, $\frac{5}{1}$ (for example) should be written as just 5.*

1. $\dfrac{0.4}{0.5}$

5. $\dfrac{0.8}{0.4}$

9. $\dfrac{0.75}{0.3}$

13. $\dfrac{300}{1.5}$

2. $\dfrac{0.6}{0.8}$

6. $\dfrac{0.35}{0.5}$

10. $\dfrac{0.95}{0.4}$

14. $\dfrac{100}{4.5}$

3. $\dfrac{0.9}{0.6}$

7. $\dfrac{0.45}{0.2}$

11. $\dfrac{200}{2.5}$

15. $\dfrac{500}{5.5}$

4. $\dfrac{0.3}{0.7}$

8. $\dfrac{0.55}{0.1}$

12. $\dfrac{100}{1.5}$

16. $\dfrac{0.09}{0.02}$

Check your answers in chapter 8.

13. ROUNDING OFF DECIMAL NUMBERS

'Rounding off' is necessary at times when liquid medication dosages are administered as drops.

ROUNDING OFF TO ONE DECIMAL PLACE

Method If the second decimal place is *5 or more*, then *add 1* to the first decimal place. If the second decimal place is *less than* 5, then *leave* the first decimal place as it is.

Example A

Write correct to one decimal place.

a. **0.62**
a. 0.6 ② ≈ 0.6

b. **1.75**
b. 1.7 ⑤ ≈ 1.8

c. **3.49**
c. 3.4 ⑨ ≈ 3.5

Note: The symbol ≈ stands for *'is approximately equal to'*.

ROUNDING OFF TO TWO DECIMAL PLACES

Method If the third decimal place is *5 or more*, then *add 1* to the second decimal place. If the third decimal place is *less than* 5, then *leave* the second decimal place as it is.

Example B

Write correct to two decimal places.

a. **0.827**
a. 0.82 ⑦ ≈ 0.83

b. **0.694**
b. 0.69 ④ ≈ 0.69

c. **2.145**
c. 2.14 ⑤ ≈ 2.15

Review exercise 2K *Rounding off*

Part i *Write each number correct to **one** decimal place.*

1. 0.93	4. 0.58	7. 2.37	10. 1.06
2. 0.47	5. 0.96	8. 1.09	11. 2.98
3. 0.85	6. 1.57	9. 0.16	12. 1.02

Part ii *Write each number correct to **two** decimal places.*

1. 0.333	4. 0.142	7. 2.714	10. 0.625
2. 1.667	5. 0.125	8. 1.285	11. 0.777
3. 0.875	6. 0.916	9. 0.636	12. 2.428

Check your answers in chapter 8.

14. FRACTION TO A DECIMAL I

⚠️ *Important:* Health professionals need to translate fractions to decimals accurately when calculating medication dosages for all forms of administration. For example, you need to know that $\frac{1}{2}$ of one litre is the same as 0.5 L, which is the same as 500 mL. Likewise, 500 mg of a medication that is supplied as 1000 mg tablets means that $\frac{1}{2}$ of that tablet is needed to administer the correct dose.

Some fractions have *exact* decimal equivalents; for example, $\frac{1}{2}$ is exactly equal to 0.5. Other fractions have only *approximate* decimal equivalents; for example, $\frac{2}{3}$ is approximately equal to 0.67. The fractions in this review exercise have *exact* decimal equivalents.

Method   Divide the numerator by the denominator.

Example A

Change $\frac{2}{5}$ to a decimal.

$5\overline{)2.0}$ ← Write as many zeros
$\underline{0.4}$ as you need

$\therefore \frac{2}{5} = 0.4$

Example B

Change $\frac{3}{8}$ to a decimal.

$8\overline{)3.0^60^40}$ ← Write as many zeros
$\underline{0.3\,7\,5}$ as you need

$\therefore \frac{3}{8} = 0.375$

Example C

Change $\frac{3}{20}$ to a decimal.

$$
\begin{array}{l}
10\overline{)3} \\
\ 2\overline{)0.3^10} \\
\ \ \ \overline{0.1\,5}
\end{array}
\quad
\begin{bmatrix}
\text{divided by 10} \\
\text{and then 2} \\
\text{since } 10 \times 2 = 20
\end{bmatrix}
\quad or \quad
\begin{aligned}
\frac{3}{20} &= \frac{15}{100} \\
&= 0.15
\end{aligned}
$$

Example D

Change $\frac{14}{25}$ to a decimal.

$$
\begin{array}{l}
5\overline{)14.^40} \\
5\overline{)2.8^30} \\
\ \ \overline{0.5\,6}
\end{array}
\quad
\begin{bmatrix}
\text{divided by 5} \\
\text{and then 5 again} \\
\text{since } 5 \times 5 = 25
\end{bmatrix}
\quad or \quad
\begin{aligned}
\frac{14}{25} &= \frac{56}{100} \\
&= 0.56
\end{aligned}
$$

Gatford and Phillips' Drug Calculations

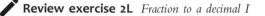

Review exercise 2L *Fraction to a decimal I*

Change each fraction to a decimal. All of these fractions have exact decimal equivalents. Refer to Examples A and B.

1. $\frac{1}{2}$ 3. $\frac{3}{4}$ 5. $\frac{3}{5}$

2. $\frac{1}{4}$ 4. $\frac{1}{5}$ 6. $\frac{7}{8}$

All of these fractions have exact decimal equivalents. Refer to Examples C and D.

7. $\frac{1}{20}$ 10. $\frac{19}{20}$ 13. $\frac{22}{25}$ 16. $\frac{27}{40}$

8. $\frac{7}{20}$ 11. $\frac{1}{25}$ 14. $\frac{1}{40}$ 17. $\frac{7}{50}$

9. $\frac{13}{20}$ 12. $\frac{8}{25}$ 15. $\frac{9}{40}$ 18. $\frac{43}{50}$

Check your answers in chapter 8.

15. FRACTION TO A DECIMAL II

The fractions in this review exercise have only approximate decimal equivalents.

Example A

Change $\frac{4}{7}$ to a decimal correct to 1 decimal place.

$$7)\overline{4.0^50} \quad \leftarrow \text{Use 2 zeros}$$
$$\underline{0.5\,\textcircled{7}} \quad \text{The second d.p. is 5 or more, therefore add 1 to the first d.p.}$$
$$\therefore \frac{4}{7} \approx 0.6$$

Example B

Change $\frac{5}{6}$ to a decimal correct to 2 decimal places.

$$6)\overline{5.0^20^20} \quad \leftarrow \text{Use 3 zeros}$$
$$\underline{0.8\,3\,\textcircled{3}} \quad \text{The third d.p. is less than 5, therefore leave second d.p. unchanged.}$$
$$\therefore \frac{5}{6} \approx 0.83$$

Example C

Change $\frac{13}{60}$ to a decimal correct to 2 decimal places.

$$10)\overline{13.0} \qquad \left[\begin{array}{l}\text{divided by 10}\\ \text{and then 6}\\ \text{since } 10\times 6 = 60\end{array}\right]$$
$$6)\overline{1.3^10^40}$$
$$\underline{0.2\,1\,\textcircled{6}}$$
$$\therefore \frac{13}{60} \approx 0.22$$

✎ Review exercise 2M *Fraction to a decimal II*

Part i *Change each fraction to a decimal correct to **one** decimal place.*

1. $\dfrac{1}{3}$

3. $\dfrac{5}{7}$

5. $\dfrac{6}{11}$

2. $\dfrac{5}{6}$

4. $\dfrac{2}{9}$

6. $\dfrac{11}{12}$

Part ii *Change each fraction to a decimal correct to **two** decimal places.*

1. $\dfrac{2}{3}$

3. $\dfrac{6}{7}$

5. $\dfrac{4}{11}$

2. $\dfrac{1}{6}$

4. $\dfrac{8}{9}$

6. $\dfrac{5}{12}$

Check your answers in chapter 8.

16. FRACTION TO A DECIMAL III

🔲 *Note:* The symbol ≈ stands for *'is approximately equal to'*.

Example A

Calculate the value of $\frac{175}{6}$ to the nearest whole number.

$$\frac{175}{6} = 175 \div 6$$

$$6 \overline{)17^55.^10}$$
$$2\,.\,9\,.\,\textcircled{1}$$

$$\therefore \frac{175}{6} \approx 29.1 \Rightarrow 29$$

If the first decimal place is *5 or more, add 1* to the whole number.

If the first decimal place is *less than 5, leave* the whole number unchanged.

Example B

Calculate the value of $\frac{7}{6}$ correct to one decimal place.

$$\frac{7}{6} = 7 \div 6$$

$$6 \overline{)7.^10^40}$$
$$1\,.\,1\,.\,\textcircled{6}$$

$$\therefore \frac{7}{6} \approx 1.16 \Rightarrow 1.2$$

If the second decimal place is *5 or more, add 1* to the first decimal place.

If the second decimal place is *less than 5, leave* the first decimal place unchanged.

Review exercise 2N *Fraction to a decimal III*

Part i *Calculate the value of each fraction to the nearest whole number. Refer to Example A.*

1. $\dfrac{100}{3}$ 4. $\dfrac{125}{4}$ 7. $\dfrac{275}{6}$ 10. $\dfrac{375}{8}$

2. $\dfrac{250}{3}$ 5. $\dfrac{72}{5}$ 8. $\dfrac{240}{7}$ 11. $\dfrac{425}{8}$

3. $\dfrac{500}{3}$ 6. $\dfrac{144}{5}$ 9. $\dfrac{300}{7}$ 12. $\dfrac{550}{9}$

Part ii *Calculate the value of each fraction correct to **one** decimal place. Refer to Example B.*

1. $\dfrac{5}{3}$ 4. $\dfrac{25}{6}$ 7. $\dfrac{50}{7}$ 10. $\dfrac{45}{8}$

2. $\dfrac{10}{3}$ 5. $\dfrac{20}{7}$ 8. $\dfrac{65}{7}$ 11. $\dfrac{70}{9}$

3. $\dfrac{35}{6}$ 6. $\dfrac{25}{7}$ 9. $\dfrac{55}{8}$ 12. $\dfrac{85}{9}$

Check your answers in chapter 8.

17. MIXED NUMBERS AND IMPROPER FRACTIONS

A *mixed number* is partly a whole number and partly a fraction: e.g., $3\frac{1}{2}$. In an *improper fraction*, the numerator is larger than the denominator: e.g., $\frac{10}{7}$.

Example A

a. **Change $\frac{17}{5}$ to a mixed number.**

$$\frac{17}{5} = 17 \div 5$$

$$= 3\frac{2}{5} \leftarrow \text{remainder}$$
$$\phantom{= 3\frac{2}{5}} \leftarrow \text{same denominator as improper fraction}$$

$$5)\overline{17}$$
$$3 + 2 \text{ remainder}$$

b. **Change $\frac{115}{4}$ to a mixed number.**

$$\frac{115}{4} = 115 \div 4$$

$$= 28\frac{3}{4} \leftarrow \text{remainder}$$
$$\phantom{= 28\frac{3}{4}} \leftarrow \text{same denominator as improper fraction}$$

$$4)\overline{115}$$
$$28 + 3 \text{ remainder}$$

Example B

a. **Change $8\frac{1}{4}$ to an improper fraction.**

$$8\frac{1}{4} = \frac{33}{4} \quad \begin{array}{l} \leftarrow 8 \times 4 + 1 = 33 \\ \leftarrow \text{same denominator as fraction in mixed number.} \end{array}$$

b. **Change $20\frac{4}{5}$ to an improper fraction.**

$$20\frac{4}{5} = \frac{104}{5} \quad \begin{array}{l} \leftarrow 20 \times 5 + 4 = 104 \\ \leftarrow \text{same denominator as fraction in mixed number.} \end{array}$$

Review exercise 20 *Mixed numbers and improper fractions*

Part i *Change these improper fractions to mixed numbers.*

1. $\dfrac{5}{2}$ 4. $\dfrac{36}{7}$ 7. $\dfrac{71}{4}$ 10. $\dfrac{101}{7}$

2. $\dfrac{11}{3}$ 5. $\dfrac{49}{9}$ 8. $\dfrac{86}{5}$ 11. $\dfrac{113}{8}$

3. $\dfrac{22}{5}$ 6. $\dfrac{65}{3}$ 9. $\dfrac{95}{6}$ 12. $\dfrac{125}{9}$

Part ii *Rewrite these mixed numbers as improper fractions.*

1. $1\frac{1}{2}$ 4. $4\frac{2}{3}$ 7. $11\frac{1}{6}$ 10. $22\frac{1}{2}$

2. $1\frac{1}{3}$ 5. $6\frac{1}{4}$ 8. $16\frac{5}{8}$ 11. $27\frac{3}{4}$

3. $2\frac{3}{5}$ 6. $9\frac{4}{5}$ 9. $17\frac{2}{9}$ 12. $32\frac{4}{7}$

Check your answers in chapter 8.

Gatford and Phillips' Drug Calculations

18. MULTIPLICATION OF FRACTIONS

There are two main methods of multiplying fractions. One method uses *cancelling before* multiplying the numerators and denominators; the other method uses *cancelling after* multiplying the numerators and denominators. We recommend the first method because this keeps the numbers smaller in working them out. Both methods are shown in Example B.

Example A

Multiply $\frac{2}{5} \times \frac{4}{7}$

Note: These fractions cannot be cancelled before multiplying.

$$\frac{2}{5} \times \frac{4}{7} = \frac{2 \times 4}{5 \times 7}$$

$$= \frac{8}{35} \left[\begin{array}{l} \text{this fraction cannot} \\ \text{be simplified} \end{array} \right]$$

Example B

Simplify $\frac{4}{9} \times \frac{21}{5}$

$$\frac{4}{\overset{3}{9}} \times \frac{\overset{7}{21}}{5} = \frac{4 \times 7}{3 \times 5}$$

note cancelling across by 3

$$= \frac{28}{15}$$

change to a mixed number

$$= 1\frac{13}{15}$$

answer may be greater than 1

$$\frac{4}{9} \times \frac{21}{5} = \frac{4 \times 21}{9 \times 5} = \frac{84}{45}$$

divide numerator and denominator by 3

$$= \frac{28}{15}$$

change to a mixed number

$$= 1\frac{13}{15}$$

answer may be greater than 1

![EXAMPLE] **Example C**

Simplify $\frac{9}{10} \times \frac{8}{15}$

$$\frac{\overset{3}{\cancel{9}}}{\underset{5}{\cancel{10}}} \times \frac{\overset{4}{\cancel{8}}}{\underset{5}{\cancel{15}}} = \frac{3 \times 4}{5 \times 5} \quad \left[\begin{array}{l}\text{note cancelling across} \\ \text{by 3 and by 2}\end{array}\right]$$

$$= \frac{12}{25} \quad 2$$

✏ Review exercise 2P *Multiplication of fractions*

Multiply these fractions. Simplify your answer where possible.

1. $\dfrac{1}{2} \times \dfrac{2}{5}$

5. $\dfrac{4}{5} \times \dfrac{25}{24}$

9. $\dfrac{6}{7} \times \dfrac{5}{24}$

2. $\dfrac{2}{3} \times \dfrac{5}{6}$

6. $\dfrac{5}{6} \times \dfrac{8}{15}$

10. $\dfrac{3}{8} \times \dfrac{12}{5}$

3. $\dfrac{3}{4} \times \dfrac{20}{9}$

7. $\dfrac{2}{7} \times \dfrac{11}{12}$

11. $\dfrac{2}{9} \times \dfrac{7}{4}$

4. $\dfrac{2}{5} \times \dfrac{3}{2}$

8. $\dfrac{4}{7} \times \dfrac{5}{3}$

12. $\dfrac{5}{9} \times \dfrac{21}{25}$

Check your answers in chapter 8.

19. MULTIPLICATION OF A FRACTION BY A WHOLE NUMBER

Example A

Multiply $\frac{5}{4} \times 6$. Simplify if possible. Write your answer as a fraction, a mixed number or a whole number.

$$\text{Simplify } \frac{5}{4} \times 6 = \frac{5}{4} \times \frac{6}{1}$$

$$= \frac{30}{4} \quad \begin{bmatrix} \text{Divide numerator and} \\ \text{denominator by 2} \end{bmatrix}$$

$$= \frac{15}{2} \quad \begin{bmatrix} \text{Change to a} \\ \text{mixed number} \end{bmatrix}$$

$$= 7\frac{1}{2}$$

Example B

Multiply $\frac{150}{125} \times 2$. Write your answer as a decimal number.

$$\frac{150}{125} \times 2 = \frac{150}{125} \times \frac{2}{1}$$

$$= \frac{300}{125} \quad \begin{bmatrix} \text{Divide numerator and} \\ \text{denominator by 5} \end{bmatrix}$$

$$= \frac{60}{25} \quad \begin{bmatrix} \text{Again divide numerator and} \\ \text{denominator by 5} \end{bmatrix}$$

$$= \frac{12}{5} \quad [\text{Divide 12 by 5}]$$

$$= 2.4$$

Review exercise 2Q *Multiply these fractions and whole numbers*

Part i *Multiply. Simplify where possible. Write each answer as a fraction, a mixed number or a whole number.*

1. $\frac{3}{4} \times 5$ 5. $\frac{3}{5} \times 10$ 9. $\frac{4}{5} \times 5$

2. $\frac{2}{5} \times 3$ 6. $\frac{2}{7} \times 3$ 10. $\frac{5}{6} \times 4$

3. $\frac{2}{3} \times 6$ 7. $\frac{3}{4} \times 6$ 11. $\frac{2}{3} \times 5$

4. $\frac{5}{3} \times 4$ 8. $\frac{5}{8} \times 3$ 12. $\frac{3}{10} \times 2$

Part ii *Multiply. Write each answer as a decimal number or as a whole number, where this occurs.*

1. $\frac{7}{4} \times 2$ 5. $\frac{25}{20} \times 2$ 9. $\frac{32}{40} \times 2$

2. $\frac{6}{10} \times 2$ 6. $\frac{18}{50} \times 5$ 10. $\frac{35}{50} \times 4$

3. $\frac{3}{10} \times 2$ 7. $\frac{90}{50} \times 2$ 11. $\frac{45}{25} \times 5$

4. $\frac{7}{20} \times 2$ 8. $\frac{60}{80} \times 5$ 12. $\frac{55}{50} \times 4$

Check your answers in chapter 8.

20. 24-HOUR TIME

Example A *Convert to 24-hour time*

a **8:45 a.m.**
b **4:20 p.m.**

a   8:45 a.m. = 08:45 hrs
b   4:20 p.m. = 4:20 + 12:00 = 16:20 hrs

Note: In practice, the colons [:] are usually omitted. Thus, 08:45 hrs would simply be written as 0845 hrs, and 16:20 hrs would be written as 1620 hrs.

Example B *Convert to a.m./p.m. time*

a **1150 hrs**
b **2015 hrs**

a   1150 hrs = 11:50 a.m.
b   2015 hrs = 2015 − 1200 = 8:15 p.m.

Example C

What is the time 6 hrs after 1915 hrs on a Thursday? Give time and day.

1915 hrs + 6 hrs 00 mins = 2515 hrs

But there are only 24 hrs in a day

2515 hrs − 2400 = 0115 hrs Friday

Note: Noon = 1200 hrs; midnight = 2400 hrs.

Gatford and Phillips' Drug Calculations

✏ Review exercise 2R *24-Hour time*

Part i *Convert to 24-hour time.*

1. 9:10 a.m.
2. 8:40 p.m.
3. 2:30 a.m.
4. 11:05 a.m.
5. 4:00 a.m.
6. 3:25 p.m.
7. 12:55 p.m.
8. 1:15 p.m.
9. 6:20 a.m.
10. 5:35 p.m.
11. 7:45 a.m.
12. 10:50 p.m.

Part ii *Convert to a.m./p.m. time.*

1. 1935 hrs
2. 2230 hrs
3. 0105 hrs
4. 0200 hrs
5. 1305 hrs
6. 1745 hrs
7. 2125 hrs
8. 0640 hrs
9. 2315 hrs
10. 0510 hrs
11. 1220 hrs
12. 1450 hrs

Part iii *Calculate the finishing times. Give answers in 24-hour time and also give the day.*

1. 8 hrs after 0945 hrs Monday
2. 7 hrs after 2230 hrs Thursday
3. 10 hrs after 1015 hrs Saturday
4. 11 hrs after 1700 hrs Tuesday
5. 9 hrs after 2025 hrs Sunday
6. 12 hrs after 0640 hrs Wednesday
7. 12 hrs after 1220 hrs Friday
8. 14 hrs after 0510 hrs Thursday

Check your answers in chapter 8.

24-HOUR TIME

a.m./p.m. time	24-Hour time (hrs)	a.m./p.m. time	24-Hour time (hrs)
1 a.m.	0100	1 p.m.	1300
2 a.m.	0200	2 p.m.	1400
3 a.m.	0300	3 p.m.	1500
4 a.m.	0400	4 p.m.	1600
5 a.m.	0500	5 p.m.	1700
6 a.m.	0600	6 p.m.	1800
7 a.m.	0700	7 p.m.	1900
8 a.m.	0800	8 p.m.	2000
9 a.m.	0900	9 p.m.	2100
10 a.m.	1000	10 p.m.	2200
11 a.m.	1100	11 p.m.	2300
12 noon	1200	12 midnight	2400

Note: You may also see midnight written as 0000 hrs. One minute past midnight is 0001.

3 | Dosage calculations for solid medications

CHAPTER CONTENTS

1. INTRODUCTION

Drugs may be administered by several routes, including inhaled, topical, parenteral injection, or infusion, and orally. The first medications that nursing students usually administer to patients are by the oral route. Oral medications can be solid, liquid, gas or gel. This chapter will concentrate on calculations of solid forms of medications.

Skills covered in this chapter include the following:

- calculating the dose required for an oral medication based on the prescription.
- identifying the best combination of tablets required for specific prescriptions, so that minimum number of tablets possible are used.
- interpreting the information on a medication chart and medication labels to accurately calculate dosages.

2. WHAT YOU NEED TO KNOW

Oral medications may be in several forms (see Chapter 1). Most oral medications are solid forms such as tablets, caplets, capsules, lozenges, and wafers. Other solid forms of medications include suppositories and pessaries. Many oral medications are available in liquid form. The liquid may be syrup, an elixir, a solution or a suspension. Dosage calculations for liquid medications will be dealt with in Chapter 4, because the formula for calculating a liquid medication dose is the same whether for oral or injectable administration.

A whole tablet is *always* preferable to a broken tablet because, unless a tablet is broken exactly, the dose will not be accurate.

⚠ SAFETY MESSAGE

If it is necessary to break a tablet, caplet or capsule, check the manufacturer's guidelines or check with the pharmacist to ensure it is acceptable to do so, because some should *never* be broken. For example scored sustained release tablets can be broken to administer half of the stock strength but un-scored sustained release tablets cannot. You must confirm the safe handling of all medications with manufacturer product information.

Check that stock strength and the strength required are given in the *same* unit of weight in a particular calculation (i.e. *both* strengths in grams or milligrams or micrograms).

Check that you have used the **same unit of weight** throughout a calculation.

Are **both** weights in grams (g)?
or are **both** weights in milligrams (mg)?
or are **both** weights in micrograms?

⚠ *Important:* Before administering any medication, if in **any** doubt about the answer to a calculation, then ask a supervisor to check your calculation.

Refer to prelim page ix for explanations of abbreviations.

3. CALCULATING DOSAGES OF SOLID MEDICATIONS

Example A *How many 50 mg tablets of atenolol should be given for a dose of atenolol 75 mg?*

$$\text{Volume required} = \frac{\text{Strength required}}{\text{Stock strength}}$$

Note: In the case of tablets, 'Volume required' refers to the number of tablets needed to achieve the prescribed dose.

In the case of solid medications, the strength of the stock is the grams, milligrams or micrograms of the medication in each tablet, caplet, capsule, lozenge, wafer, pessary or suppository.

The formula can be abbreviated to the following:

$$\begin{aligned}
\text{VR} &= \frac{\text{SR}}{\text{SS}} \\
&= \frac{75 \text{ mg}}{50 \text{ mg}} \times 1 \text{ tablet} \\
&= \frac{3}{2} \text{ tablets} \\
&= 1\frac{1}{2} \text{ tablets}
\end{aligned}$$

Example B *A patient is prescribed 0.25 mg of digoxin, PO at 0800 hrs. Each digoxin tablet contains 125 micrograms of the medication. How many of these tablets should the patient receive?*

Note: First step — change both strengths to the same units.

$$0.25 \text{ mg} = 250 \text{ micrograms}$$

$$\text{Volume required} = \frac{\text{Strength required}}{\text{Stock strength}}$$

The formula can be abbreviated to the following:

$$\text{VR} = \frac{\text{SR}}{\text{SS}}$$

$$= \frac{250 \text{ micrograms}}{125 \text{ micrograms}} \times 1 \text{ tablet}$$

$$= \frac{2}{1} \text{ tablets}$$

$$= 2 \text{ tablets}$$

If you are having difficulty simplifying the fractions in these examples, then refer to Review exercises 2H and 2I in Chapter 2.

Dosage calculations for solid medications

Exercise 3A

1. A patient is prescribed rectal paracetamol 1 g. The stock available is 500 mg suppositories. Calculate the number of suppositories required.

2. Prescribed: codeine 15 mg, PO, 1200 hrs. Stock on hand: codeine 30 mg tablets. How many tablets should be administered to the patient?

3. A patient is prescribed furosemide (frusemide) 60 mg, PO. In the ward are 40 mg tablets. How many tablets should be given?

4. How many 300 mg caplets of ibuprofen are needed for a dose of 0.6 g?

5. 750 mg of ciprofloxacin is required. The available capsules are of strength 500 mg. How many capsules should be given?

6. A patient is prescribed 150 mg of enteric–coated aspirin at 1000 hrs. On hand are 300 mg scored sustained release tablets. What number should be given?

7. 450 mg of fentanyl is prescribed. Stock available is 300 mg lozenges. How many lozenges should the patient receive?

8. 25 micrograms estradiol pessary is prescribed. How many 50 micrograms pessary tablets should be given?

9. The stock available in the unit is diazepam 5 mg tablets. How many tablets are to be administered if the prescription is diazepam 12.5 mg at 1400 hrs?

10. Digoxin 125 micrograms is prescribed at 0800 hrs. Tablets available are 0.25 mg. How many tablets should be given?

11. Glycerol trinitrate is available in 300 micrograms tablets for sub-lingual administration. The patient is instructed to place one tablet under their tongue when experiencing angina and if the pain persists after 5 min to take another sub-lingual tablet. How many milligrams of glycerol trinitrate will be administered in two doses?

12. The maximum dose of paracetamol is 4 g in 24 hrs. The tablets supplied are 500 mg paracetamol. How many tablets can be safely administered in 1 day?

Check your answers in chapter 8.

13. A patient is prescribed ondansetron wafer 8 mg, PO at 1700 hrs. In the ward are 4 mg wafers. What number should be given?

14. 12.5 mg of captopril is prescribed for hypertension. On hand are tablets with a strength of 25 mg. How many tablets should be given?

15. How many 30 mg tablets of codeine should be given for a prescription of codeine 45 mg?

Check your answers in chapter 8.

4. COMBINATIONS OF TABLETS

For some medications, tablets are available in several strengths. The tablets may be coloured or imprinted differently to differentiate them and reduce the risk of error when dispensing.

Note: The *least* number of tablets should be chosen as the best combination to be administered. Administering the correct dose using the fewest tablets enhances the comfort and convenience for the patient as well as contributing to their adherence with the treatment regimen.

Example *Choose the best combination of 1 mg, 2 mg, 5 mg or 10 mg tablets of warfarin for each dosage.*

The number of tablets should be as few as possible and only whole tablets may be used.

a. **6 mg**   b. **8 mg**   c. **11 mg**   d. **14 mg**

a. 5 mg + 1 mg (2 tablets)
b. 5 mg + 2 mg + 1 mg (3 tablets)
c. 10 mg + 1 mg (2 tablets)
d. 10 mg + 2 mg + 2 mg (3 tablets)

Exercise 3B *Choose the best combination of **whole** tablets for each prescription.*

The number of tablets should be as few as possible.

1. *Prescribed*: warfarin tablets
   Strengths available: 1 mg, 2 mg, 5 mg and 10 mg
   Dosages required: a. 4 mg b. 9 mg c. 12 mg d. 15 mg

2. *Prescribed*: diazepam tablets
   Strengths available: 2 mg, 5 mg and 10 mg
   Dosages required: a. 7 mg b. 9 mg c. 15 mg d. 20 mg

3. *Prescribed*: verapamil tablets
   Strengths available: 40 mg, 80 mg, 120 mg and 160 mg
   Dosages required: a. 200 mg b. 240 mg c. 280 mg d. 320 mg

4. *Prescribed*: prazosin tablets
   Strengths available: 1 mg, 2 mg and 5 mg
   Dosages required: a. 6 mg b. 8 mg c. 9 mg d. 11 mg

5. *Prescribed*: furosemide (frusemide) tablets
   Strengths available: 20 mg, 40 mg, 80 mg and 500 mg
   Dosages required: a. 60 mg b. 100 mg c. 200 mg d. 560 mg

6. *Prescribed*: thioridazine tablets
   Strengths available: 10 mg, 25 mg, 50 mg and 100 mg
   Dosages required: a. 35 mg b. 60 mg c. 75 mg d. 120 mg

7. *Prescribed:* warfarin tablets
   Strengths available: 1 mg, 2 mg, 5 mg and 10 mg
   Dosage required: a. 3 mg b. 7 mg c. 13 mg d. 16 mg

8. *Prescribed:* prednisolone tablets
   Strength available: 1 mg, 5 mg and 10 mg
   Dosage required: a. 15 mg b. 20 mg c. 26 mg d. 35 mg

9. *Prescribed:* diclofenac potassium tablets
   Strength available: 25 mg and 50 mg
   Dosage required: a. 50 mg b. 75 mg c. 125 mg d. 150 mg

Check your answers in chapter 8.

10. *Prescribed:* ciprofloxacin tablets
    Strength available: 100 mg, 250 mg and 500 mg
    Dosage required: a. 250 mg   b. 400 mg   c. 600 mg   d. 750 mg

11. *Prescribed:* atenolol
    Strength available: 25 mg and 50 mg
    Dosage required: a. 75 mg   b. 100 mg   c. 125 mg   d. 200 mg

12. *Prescribed:* furosemide tablets
    Strength available: 20 mg and 40 mg
    Dosage required: a. 60 mg   b. 80 mg   c. 100 mg   d. 120 mg

Check your answers in chapter 8.

5. CALCULATIONS OF SOLID ORAL MEDICATIONS INVOLVING PRESCRIPTIONS AND MEDICATION LABELS

Exercise 3C *Read each prescription and medication label carefully.*

1. A patient is to be given their daily morning dose of oral ramipril. How many of these Tritace tablets should be given?

Regular medicines

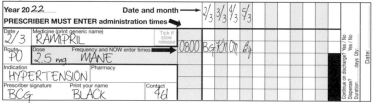

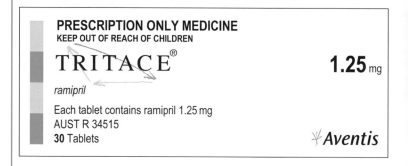

PRESCRIPTION ONLY MEDICINE
KEEP OUT OF REACH OF CHILDREN

TRITACE®

1.25 mg

ramipril

Each tablet contains ramipril 1.25 mg
AUST R 34515
30 Tablets

⚜*Aventis*

Check your answers in chapter 8.

2. How many Metronide tablets should be given for a dose in the following prescription of oral metronidazole?

Regular medicines

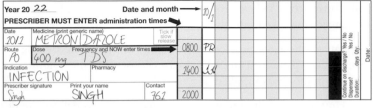

Year 20 22		Date and month ➤		10/1													
PRESCRIBER MUST ENTER administration times ➤																	
Date 20/1	Medicine (print generic name) METRONIDAZOLE		Tick if slow release	0800	PR										Continue on discharge? Yes / No	
Route PO	Dose 400 mg	Frequency and NOW enter times ➤ TDS		1400	11										Dispense? Yes / No days Qty:	Date:
Indication INFECTION		Pharmacy		1400	11											
Prescriber signature Singh	Print your name SINGH		Contact 761	2000											Duration:	

PRESCRIPTION ONLY MEDICINE
KEEP OUT OF REACH OF CHILDREN

METRONIDE® 200

Metronidazole Tablets
21 TABLETS
Each tablet contains METRONIDAZOLE 200 mg
AUST R 65540

Check your answers in chapter 8.

6. CASE SCENARIO

Greg is a 52-year-old male with aggressive prostate cancer. Greg had a laparoscopic radical prostatectomy 1 month ago. He has been discharged home and into the care of his general practitioner.

To manage the acute post-operative pain, the anaesthetic treating team initially prescribed an oral opioid analgesic of 10 mg 4 hourly. The medication was supplied as 5 mg tablets.

1. How many of the supplied tablets are needed to deliver the dose prescribed?

    This analgesic medication can be titrated up to 15 mg 4 hourly to manage breakthrough pain. Greg remains in pain, and so, the treating doctor increases the next due dose to 15 mg of the same opioid analgesia. You are a community nurse.

2. How many tablets of the medication will you administer in the next due dose?

    Since the surgery, Greg is also prescribed an anti-androgen medication. The anti-androgen tablet supplied for Greg has 50 mg of medication per tablet. The prescribed dose is 100 mg mane.

3. How may tablets should Greg take each morning?

    Greg had chemotherapy after the surgery. He experienced chemotherapy-induced nausea. He was prescribed a 5HT$_3$ antagonist to prevent the nausea and vomiting. The medication is available as 2 mg, 1 mg and 5 mg tablets. The dose prescribed is 2.5 mg daily.

4. Which tablet/s will you use to administer the correct dose using the least number of tablets?

    Greg experienced significant weight loss, and his nausea and vomiting are concerning to the general practitioner because poor nutrition contributes to extended recovery from surgery. Therefore, the general practitioner prescribes the following oral nutritional supplements:

    Thiamine hydrochloride 100 mg daily in two divided doses.

    Pyridoxine 240 mg by sustained release caplet daily.

    The community pharmacy supplies the thiamine hydrochloride as 50 mg tablets. The pyridoxine is a 240 mg sustained release caplet.

5. How many thiamine tablets should Greg take at one time?
6. How many times in one day will he take the pyridoxine?

Greg's pain remains unmanaged and he is having trouble swallowing the medications. So, the general practitioner decides to alter the oral form of the opioid to a transdermal patch for sustained management of the pain.

Pain management protocols suggest a step–wise approach and to commence the new medication at 50% of the equianalgesic dose and titrate to the maximum dose (NPS MedicineWise 2020). Opioid equivalence charts, for example, Table 3.1, recommend equivalence ranges to guide the prescribers (Gloucestershire Hospitals 2020).

TABLE 3.1 Fentanyl transdermal dose recommendations.

24-hour oral morphine dose mg/day (range)	Equivalent fentanyl patch micrograms/hour
30	12
60 (45–89)	25
90	37
120 (90–149)	50
150	62
180 (150–209)	75
240 (210–269)	100
300 (270–329)	125
360 (330–389)	150
420 (390–449)	175
480 (450–509)	200
540 (510–569)	225
600 (570–629)	250
660 (630–689)	275
720 (690–749)	300

The transdermal opioid is available as 12.5, 25, 50, 75 or 100 micrograms/hr patches.

7. What opioid patch would be the best for the pharmacist supply for Greg's initial dose? (see Table 3.1 showing therapeutic ranges.)

Please refer to local drug monographs and protocols to check the dosages and equivalences in question 7 to ensure patient safety.

For ease of administration for Greg, the general practitioner changed the oral antiemetic prescription from a tablet to a wafer. Ondansetron 4 mg wafers are supplied by the pharmacy.

8. If the order is for 8 mg ondansetron twice daily, how many wafers will be used in 24 hrs?

Greg has become constipated as an adverse effect of some medications. Bisacodyl enteric-coated tablets are prescribed for morning administration along with a 10 mg suppository for 1830 hrs daily. The bisacodyl tablets contain 5 mg of the medication.

9. How many tablets will you give if the order is for 10 mg mane?

10. Using an analogue clock, what time of the day is the suppository due?

References

Gloucestershire Hospitals 2020, Opioid Equivalence Chart. Available at https://www.gloshospitals.nhs.uk/gps/treatment-guidelines/opioid-equivalence-chart/.

NPS MedicineWise 2020, Fentanyl patches (Durogesic) for chronic pain. Available at https://www.nps.org.au/radar/articles/fentanyl-patches-durogesic-for-chronic-pain.

4 | Dosage calculations for liquid medications

CHAPTER CONTENTS

1. INTRODUCTION

Correct measurement of dosages of liquid medications is essential. An overdose can be dangerous; too low a dose may result in a medication being ineffective. If the dose is too high it will be an overdose and could result in harm, injury or death.

In this chapter, you will be shown how to calculate the volume of liquid medication to be drawn up in a syringe or measured in a medicine cup. The focus of this chapter is on oral and injectable liquid dosages.

 SAFETY MESSAGES

Liquid medications for oral administration can never be injected. However, some liquid medications for injection can be ingested. You must know the correct route for administration.

⚠ *Important:* Oral liquid suspensions must be shaken thoroughly before measuring the required volume. Be aware to follow the manufacturer and local policy guidelines for the expiry date of re-constituted medications once they are opened. Also note the appropriate method of storage once the medication has been opened. For example, most medications can be stored in a cool dry place below 25 degrees unless refrigeration is required (usually between 2 and 8 degrees).

Administering medications by injection can be lethal and fatal if the medication dosage calculation is incorrect. The risk is greater with injectable medications because they are usually absorbed faster than other routes of administration. For example, injecting a medication directly into the blood stream will have a more prompt and potent effect. Therefore, when calculating medication dosages for injection, you must check and confirm your arithmetic before commencing administration. You must also understand the prescription that denotes the strength of medication required as well as the labelling on the medication that indicates the amount of the medication relative to the volume of stock liquid.

2. WHAT YOU NEED TO KNOW

The number of decimal places in each answer should relate to the graduations on the syringe being used to administer the medication. Syringes with a capacity of more than 1 mL are usually graduated in tenths or fifths of a millilitre: so, for volumes *greater than* 1 mL, calculate answers to *one* decimal place. Syringes with a capacity of 1 mL or less are often graduated in hundredths of a millilitre: so, for volumes *less than* 1 mL, calculate answers to *two* decimal places.

Remember the following:

- Give answers greater than 1 mL correct to one decimal place.
- Give answers less than 1 mL correct to two decimal places.
- If the next decimal place is five or more, add one to the previous digit.
- Check that stock strength and the strength required are given in the *same* units in a particular calculation (i.e., *both* strengths in grams or milligrams or micrograms).

⚠ *Important:* If in **any** doubt about the answer to a calculation, then ask a supervisor to check your work.

Refer to prelim page ix for explanations of abbreviations in these exercises.

3. STRENGTH OF SOLUTION ACCORDING TO VOLUME

Example for oral administration *A syrup for oral administration contains penicillin 125 mg/5 mL.* How many milligrams of penicillin are in the following volumes of the syrup?*

a. **10 mL**   b. **15 mL**   c. **25 mL**

a. Each 5 mL contains 125 mg penicillin

$$10 \text{ mL} \div 5 \text{ mL} = 2$$

$$2 \times 125 \text{ mg} = 250 \text{ mg penicillin}$$

b. Each 5 mL contains 125 mg penicillin

$$15 \text{ mL} \div 5 \text{ mL} = 3$$

$$3 \times 125 \text{ mg} = 375 \text{ mg penicillin}$$

c. Each 5 mL contains 125 mg penicillin

$$25 \text{ mL} \div 5 \text{ mL} = 5$$

$$5 \times 125 \text{ mg} = 625 \text{ mg penicillin}$$

*Note: 125 mg/5 mL means 125 mg per 5 mL.

Example for intravenous administration *A solution for injection contains heparin 5000 units/5 mL. How many units of heparin are in the following volumes of solution for injection?*

a. 6 mL   b. 8 mL   c. 10 mL

a. Each 5 mL contains 5000 units of heparin

$$6 \text{ mL} \div 5 \text{ mL} = 1.2$$

$$1.2 \times 5000 \text{ units} = 6000 \text{ units}$$

b. Each 5 mL contains 5000 units of heparin

$$8 \text{ mL} \div 5 \text{ mL} = 1.6$$

$$1.6 \times 5000 \text{ units} = 8000 \text{ units}$$

c. Each 5 mL contains 5000 units of heparin

$$10 \text{ mL} \div 5 \text{ mL} = 2$$

$$2 \times 5000 \text{ units} = 10{,}000 \text{ units}$$

Dosage calculations for liquid medications

🖊 Exercise 4A

1. An injectable solution contains furosemide (frusemide) 10 mg/1 mL. How many milligrams of frusemide are in
   a. 2 mL   b. 3 mL   c. 5 mL of the solution?

2. A solution for injection contains morphine hydrochloride 2 mg/mL. How many milligrams of morphine hydrochloride are in
   a. 3 mL   b. 5 mL   c. 7 mL of the solution?

3. A solution of morphine hydrochloride for injection contains 40 mg/mL. How many milligrams of morphine hydrochloride are in
   a. 2 mL   b. 5 mL   c. 10 mL of this solution?

4. An oral suspension contains phenytoin 125 mg/5 mL. How many milligrams of phenytoin are in
   a. 20 mL   b. 30 mL   c. 40 mL of the suspension?

5. An injection solution contains magnesium 20 mg/5 mL. How many milligrams of fluoxetine are in
   a. 10 mL   b. 25 mL   c. 40 mL of the solution?

6. An oral suspension contains erythromycin 250 mg/5 mL. How many milligrams of erythromycin are in
   a. 10 mL   b. 20 mL   c. 30 mL of the suspension?

7. A syrup for oral administration contains chlorpromazine 25 mg/5 mL. How many milligrams of chlorpromazine are in
   a. 10 mL   b. 30 mL   c. 50 mL of the syrup?

8. A mixture for ingestion contains penicillin 250 mg/5 mL. How many milligrams of penicillin are in
   a. 15 mL   b. 25 mL   c. 35 mL of the mixture?

Check your answers in chapter 8.

9. An injectable solution contains clonazepam 10 mg/mL. How many milligrams of clonazepam are in
   a. 5 mL   b. 10 mL   c. 25 mL of the solution?

10. An oral suspension contains erythromycin 250 mg/5 mL. How many milligrams of erythromycin are in
   a. 15 mL   b. 25 mL   c. 35 mL of the suspension?

Check your answers in chapter 8.

4. ESTIMATING THE VOLUME FOR INJECTION

It is important to learn how to estimate an answer *before* beginning
to work out the actual answer so that you have a sense of what is
accurate.

Example A *Pethidine 75 mg is to be given by intramuscular (IM)
injection. Stock ampoules of pethidine contain 100 mg in 2 mL. Is the volume to
be drawn up for injection equal to 2 mL, less than 2 mL or more than 2 mL?*

You will confirm your estimation by performing the calculation below:

A stock ampoule contains 100 mg of pethidine.
Volume of ampoule = 2 mL
75 mg (prescribed) is *less than* 100 mg (ampoule).
Therefore, volume to be drawn up is *less than* 2 mL.

Example B *Vancomycin 1200 mg is prescribed at 2400 hrs. Stock vials
contain vancomycin 1 g in 10 mL (once diluted). Is the volume of stock required
for injection equal to 10 mL, less than 10 mL or more than 10 mL?*

A stock vial contains 1 g of vancomycin.
1 g = 1 gram = 1000 mg
Volume of vial = 10 mL
1200 mg (prescribed) is *more than* 1000 mg (vial).
Therefore, volume required is *more than* 10 mL.

Example C *A patient is to be given 12,000 units of Calciparin at 0600 hrs. Available ampoules contain 25,000 units in 1 mL. Should the volume to be drawn up for injection be equal to 1 mL, less than 1 mL or more than 1 mL?*

A stock ampoule contains 25,000 units.
Volume of ampoule = 1 mL.
12,000 units (prescribed) is *less than* 25,000 units (ampoule).
Therefore, volume to be drawn up is *less than* 1 mL.

⚠ *Important:* Think about each answer. Does it make sense? Is the dose or volume too large for the type of injection or medication prescribed?

Exercise 4B *Choose the correct answer to each problem.*

The answer will be equal to, less than or more than the volume of the stock ampoule or vial.

1. An injection of morphine 9 mg is prescribed. A stock ampoule contains morphine 15 mg in 1 mL. The volume to be drawn up for injection will be equal to 1 mL/less than 1 mL/more than 1 mL.

2. A patient is to receive an injection of ondansetron 6 mg. Stock ampoules contain ondansetron 4 mg in 2 mL. The volume to be drawn up for injection is equal to 2 mL/less than 2 mL/more than 2 mL.

3. Furosemide (frusemide) 80 mg is prescribed. Ampoules contain furosemide 250 mg/5 mL. The volume required for injection is: equal to 5 mL/less than 5 mL/more than 5 mL.

4. Benzylpenicillin 1.2 g is prescribed. Stock vials contain 600 mg in 2 mL, when diluted. The volume of stock required is equal to 2 mL/less than 2 mL/more than 2 mL.

5. A patient is prescribed flucloxacillin 1000 mg, intravenous (IV). If stock ampoules contain 1 g in 10 mL, once diluted, then the amount of stock solution to be drawn up will be equal to 10 mL/less than 10 mL/more than 10 mL.

6. On hand are digoxin ampoules containing 500 micrograms in 2 mL. An injection of 225 micrograms is prescribed. The volume required is equal to 2 mL/less than 2 mL/more than 2 mL.

7. Heparin is available at a strength of 1000 units/mL. The volume needed to give 1250 units is equal to 1 mL/less than 1 mL/more than 1 mL.

Think carefully about each answer in the exercises that follow in this chapter. Should the volume drawn up for the injection be equal to, less than or more than the volume of the stock ampoule?

Check your answers in chapter 8.

5. CALCULATING VOLUMES OF DOSAGES FOR INJECTION

Medications for injection are in the form of liquids or powder for reconstitution into liquid. Therefore, the medication dosage calculations will be expressed in millilitres. However, the medication strengths are expressed in milligrams and can differ depending on the strength of the medication stock. You will need to calculate the milligrams required and also the volume of the stock solution required to achieve the correct dose or prescribed medication expressed as milligrams per millilitre.

Example A *A patient is prescribed furosemide (frusemide) 60 mg, IV. Ampoules contain furosemide 80 mg in 2 mL. Calculate the volume required for injection.*

$$\text{Volume required} = \frac{\text{Strength required}}{\text{Stock strength}} \times [\text{Volume of stock solution}]$$

$$= \frac{60 \text{ mg}}{80 \text{ mg}} \times 2 \text{ mL}$$

$$= \frac{60}{80} \times \frac{2}{1} \text{ mL}$$

$$= \frac{3}{2} \text{ mL}$$

$$= 1.5 \text{ mL}$$

Dosage calculations for liquid medications

Example B *An injection of digoxin 175 micrograms is prescribed. Stock on hand is digoxin 500 micrograms in 2 mL. What volume of stock solution should be given?*

The *volume required* formula can be abbreviated to the following:

$$VR = \frac{SR}{SS} \times VS$$

$$= \frac{175 \quad \text{micrograms}}{500 \quad \text{micrograms}} \times 2\ \text{mL}$$

$$= \frac{175}{500} \times \frac{2}{1}\ \text{mL}$$

$$= \frac{7}{10}\ \text{mL}$$

$$= 0.7\ \text{mL}$$

If you are having difficulty simplifying these fractions, then refer to Review exercises 2H and 2I in Chapter 2.

Exercise 4C

1. An injection of morphine 8 mg is required. Ampoules on hand contain 10 mg in 1 mL. What volume should be drawn up for injection?

2. Digoxin ampoules on hand contain 500 micrograms in 2 mL. What volume is needed to administer 350 micrograms?

3. A child is prescribed 9 mg of gentamicin by IM injection at 0900 hrs. Stock ampoules contain 20 mg in 2 mL. What volume is needed for the injection?

4. Pethidine 85 mg is to be given IM. Stock ampoules contain pethidine 100 mg in 2 mL. Calculate the volume of stock required.

5. A patient is to receive an injection of gentamicin 60 mg IM at 0200 hrs. Ampoules on hand contain 80 mg/2 mL. Calculate the volume required.

6. A patient is prescribed naloxone 0.6 mg IV immediately (stat). Stock ampoules contain 0.4 mg/2 mL. What volume should be drawn up for injection?

Check your answers in chapter 8.

Dosage calculations for liquid medications

✎ **Exercise 4D**

1. Vancomycin 500 mg is prescribed at 2000 hrs. Stock on hand contains 1 g in 10 mL, once diluted. What volume is required?

2. A patient is to receive an IV dose of gentamicin 160 mg. Stock ampoules contain 100 mg in 2 mL. Calculate the volume to be drawn up for injection.

3. How much morphine solution must be withdrawn for a 7.5 mg dose if a stock ampoule contains 15 mg in 1 mL?

4. A patient is prescribed 200 mg of furosemide (frusemide) at 1000 hrs. Stock is 250 mg in 5 mL. Calculate the volume that is needed for injection.

5. Heparin is available at a strength of 5000 units/5 mL. What volume is needed to give 800 units?

6. Phenobarbitone 40 mg has been prescribed. Stock ampoules contain 200 mg/mL. What volume should be given?

7. A patient is prescribed pethidine 65 mg stat. Stock ampoules of pethidine contain 100 mg in 2 mL. Calculate the volume to be drawn up for injection.

8. A patient is to be given ranitidine 40 mg IV at 1230 hrs. Stock ampoules have a strength of 50 mg/2 mL. What volume of stock should be injected?

9. Morphine 5.5 mg at 1600 hrs is prescribed. Stock ampoules contain 10 mg/mL. What volume should be drawn up for injection?

10. A patient is to be given flucloxacillin 250 mg by injection. Stock vials contain 1 g in 10 mL, after dilution. Calculate the required volume.

11. Stock heparin has a strength of 5000 units/mL. What volume must be drawn up to give 6500 units subcut?

Check your answers in chapter 8.

93

Calculate the volume of stock to be drawn up for injection

12. Pethidine 60 mg stat is prescribed. Stock ampoules contain 100 mg in 2 mL.

13. An adult is prescribed metoclopramide 15 mg, for nausea. On hand are ampoules containing 10 mg/mL.

14. A patient is prescribed erythromycin 250 mg IV at 1430 hrs. Stock on hand contains 1 g in 10 mL, once diluted.

15. Tramadol hydrochloride 80 mg is required. Available stock contains 100 mg in 2 mL.

16. A patient is prescribed benzylpenicillin 800 mg at 0830 hrs. On hand is benzylpenicillin 1.2 g in 6 mL.

17. An adult patient with tuberculosis is to be given 500 mg of capreomycin every second day by IM injection. Stock on hand contains 1 g in 3 mL.

18. Digoxin ampoules on hand contain 500 micrograms in 2 mL. Digoxin 150 micrograms is prescribed.

19. Stock Calciparin contains 25,000 units in 1 mL. 15,000 units of Calciparin is prescribed.

20. Penicillin 450 mg at 2000 hrs is prescribed. Stock ampoules contain 600 mg in 5 mL.

Check your answers in chapter 8.

Dosage calculations for liquid medications

✎ **Exercise 4E** *Calculate the volume of stock solution to be drawn up for injection.*

Give answers greater than 1 mL correct to one decimal place and answers less than 1 mL correct to two decimal places. If the next decimal place is five or more, add one to the previous digit.

1. *Prescribed:* erythromycin 200 mg
   Stock: 300 mg in 10 mL

2. *Prescribed:* morphine 20 mg
   Stock: 15 mg in 1 mL

3. *Prescribed:* atropine 0.5 mg
   Stock: 0.6 mg in 1 mL

4. *Prescribed:* atropine 800 micrograms
   Stock: 1.2 mg in 1 mL

5. *Prescribed:* naloxone 0.35 mg
   Stock: 0.4 mg/mL

6. *Prescribed:* capreomycin 850 mg
   Stock: 2 g/mL

7. *Prescribed:* metoclopramide 7 mg
   Stock: 10 mg/2 mL

8. *Prescribed:* heparin 1750 units
   Stock: 1000 units/mL

9. *Prescribed:* buscopan 0.25 mg
   Stock: 0.4 mg/2 mL

If you are having difficulty with rounding off decimal answers, then refer to Review exercise 2K in Chapter 2.

Check your answers in chapter 8.

Exercise 4F *Calculate the volume of stock required. Give answers greater than 1 mL correct to one decimal place and answers less than 1 mL correct to two decimal places.*

Prescribed	Dosage	Stock ampoule
1. Morphine	12 mg	15 mg/mL
2. Calciparin	7000 units	25,000 units in 1 mL
3. Benzylpenicillin	1500 mg	1.2 g in 10 mL
4. Heparin	3000 units	5000 units/mL
5. Phenobarbitone	70 mg	200 mg/mL
6. Pethidine	80 mg	100 mg in 2 mL
7. Buscopan	0.24 mg	0.4 mg/2 mL
8. Digoxin	200 micrograms	500 micrograms in 2 mL
9. Furosemide (frusemide)	150 mg	250 mg in 5 mL
10. Ondansetron	5 mg	4 mg in 2 mL
11. Capreomycin	800 mg	1 g in 5 mL
12. Tramadol	120 mg	100 mg in 2 mL
13. Gentamicin	70 mg	80 mg in 2 mL
14. Vancomycin	750 mg	1 g in 5 mL
15. Morphine	7.5 mg	10 mg in 1 mL
16. Ceftriaxone	1250 mg	1 g/3 mL
17. Buscopan	25 mg	20 mg in 1 mL
18. Dexamethasone	3 mg	4 mg/mL
19. Vancomycin	1.2 g	1000 mg/5 mL
20. Naloxone	0.5 mg	0.4 mg/mL

Check your answers in chapter 8.

6. CALCULATING VOLUMES OF DOSAGES FOR INGESTION

Example A *750 mg of erythromycin is to be given orally at 0700 hrs. Stock suspension contains 250 mg/5 mL. Calculate the volume to be given.*

$$\text{Volume required} = \frac{\text{Strength required}}{\text{Stock strength}} \times [\text{Volume of stock solution}]$$

$$= \frac{750 \text{ mg}}{250 \text{ mg}} \times 5 \text{ mL}$$

$$= \frac{750}{250} \times \frac{5}{1} \text{ mL}$$

$$= \frac{3}{1} \times \frac{5}{1} \text{ mL} \left[\text{after simplifying} \frac{750}{250} \right]$$

$$= 15 \text{ mL}$$

Example B *A patient is prescribed 800 mg of penicillin, orally (PO). The stock available in the unit has a strength of 250 mg/5 mL. Calculate the volume required.*

The *volume required* formula can be abbreviated to the following:

$$\text{VR} = \frac{\text{SR}}{\text{SS}} \times \text{VS}$$

$$= \frac{800 \text{ mg}}{250 \text{ mg}} \times 5 \text{ mL}$$

$$= \frac{800}{250} \times \frac{5}{1} \text{ mL}$$

$$= \frac{16}{5} \times \frac{5}{1} \text{ mL} \left[\text{after simplifying} \frac{800}{250} \right]$$

$$= 16 \text{ mL}$$

If you are having difficulty simplifying the fractions in these examples, then refer to Review exercises 2H and 2I in Chapter 2.

Exercise 4G *You are given the prescribed dosage and the strength of stock available. Calculate the volume to be given.*

1. *Prescribed:* penicillin 500 mg
   Available: syrup 125 mg/5 mL

2. *Prescribed:* furosemide (frusemide) 40 mg
   Available: solution 10 mg/mL

3. *Prescribed:* morphine hydrochloride 100 mg
   Available: solution 40 mg/mL

4. *Prescribed:* paracetamol 180 mg
   Available: suspension 120 mg/5 mL

5. *Prescribed:* phenytoin 150 mg
   Available: solution 125 mg/5 mL

6. *Prescribed:* erythromycin 1250 mg
   Available: suspension 250 mg/5 mL

7. *Prescribed:* fluoxetine 30 mg
   Available: solution 20 mg/5 mL

8. *Prescribed:* penicillin 1000 mg
   Available: mixture 250 mg/5 mL

9. *Prescribed:* chlorpromazine 35 mg
   Available: syrup 25 mg/5 mL

10. *Prescribed:* penicillin 1200 mg
    Available: mixture 250 mg/5 mL

11. A patient is prescribed 750 mg of erythromycin, orally. Calculate the volume required if the suspension on hand has a strength of 250 mg/5 mL.

12. Paracetamol 750 mg is to be given at 1500 hrs as a syrup. The available stock contains 150 mg/5 mL. Calculate the volume of syrup to be given.

13. A patient is prescribed penicillin 400 mg, orally, at 1600 hrs. Stock syrup has a strength of 125 mg/5 mL. What volume should be given?

Check your answers in chapter 8.

14. Flucloxacillin 375 mg is prescribed. Stock solution contains 125 mg/5 mL. What volume should the patient be given?

15. Furosemide (frusemide) 125 mg at 0200 hrs is prescribed. Stock solution is 50 mg/mL. What volume of solution should be given?

Check your answers in chapter 8.

7. CALCULATIONS FOR ORAL LIQUID MEDICATIONS INVOLVING PRESCRIPTIONS AND MEDICATION LABELS

✏ **Exercise 4H** *Read each prescription and medication label carefully. Each medication label refers to the stock available in the ward. Calculate the volume to be drawn up in the syringe.*

1. a. Using the medication label below, calculate how many milligrams of furosemide (frusemide) are in
   i. 1 mL
   ii. 2 mL

PRESCRIPTION ONLY MEDICINE
KEEP OUT OF REACH OF CHILDREN

Lasix® Oral Solution

Each mL contains
10 mg of Frusemide
Also contains
methyl hydroxybenzoate
30 mL

005548

Lasix®
This product is filled under nitrogen. Use within three weeks of opening. Protect from light. **Store at 2°C to 8°C.** (Refrigerate. Do not freeze.)
Aventis Pharma Pty Ltd
27 Sirius Road
Lane Cove NSW 2066
Aventis Pharma Limited
Auckland New Zealand

⚘*Aventis*

   b. Calculate the volume required for the dose in the prescription.

Regular medicines

Year 20 22		Date and month ⟶		4/2								
PRESCRIBER MUST ENTER administration times ⟶												
Date 4/2	Medicine (print generic name) FRUSEMIDE	Tick if slow release										Yes / No
Route PO	Dose 40 mg	Frequency and NOW enter times ⟶ MANE	0800									Yes / No
Indication HEART FAILURE		Pharmacy LIQUID										
Prescriber signature NwG	Print your name NwOJU	Contact 961										

Check your answers in chapter 8.

2. a. Using the medication label below, calculate how many milligrams of chlorpromazine are in
   i. 5 mL
   ii. 10 mL

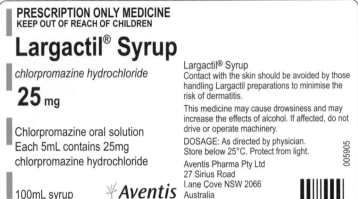

PRESCRIPTION ONLY MEDICINE
KEEP OUT OF REACH OF CHILDREN

Largactil® Syrup

chlorpromazine hydrochloride

25 mg

Chlorpromazine oral solution
Each 5mL contains 25mg
chlorpromazine hydrochloride

100mL syrup ✴Aventis

Largactil® Syrup
Contact with the skin should be avoided by those handling Largactil preparations to minimise the risk of dermatitis.

This medicine may cause drowsiness and may increase the effects of alcohol. If affected, do not drive or operate machinery.

DOSAGE: As directed by physician.
Store below 25°C. Protect from light.

Aventis Pharma Pty Ltd
27 Sirius Road
Lane Cove NSW 2066
Australia

005905

b. Calculate the volume required for one prescribed dose.

Regular medicines

Year 20 22	Date and month ➞		15/1											
PRESCRIBER MUST ENTER administration times ➞														

Date 15/1	Medicine (print generic name) CHLORPROMAZINE	Tick if slow release	0800						Continue on discharge? Yes / No
Route Po	Dose 40 mg	Frequency and NOW enter times TDS	1400						Dispense? Yes / No
Indication AGITATION	Pharmacy LIQUID								days Qty:
Prescriber signature TZowski	Print your name ZOWSKI	Contact 588	2000						Duration: Date:

Check your answers in chapter 8.

8. CALCULATIONS FOR INJECTABLE LIQUID MEDICATIONS INVOLVING PRESCRIPTIONS AND MEDICATION LABELS

Exercise 4I *Read each prescription and medication label carefully. Each medication label refers to the stock available in the ward. Calculate the volume to be drawn up in the syringe.*

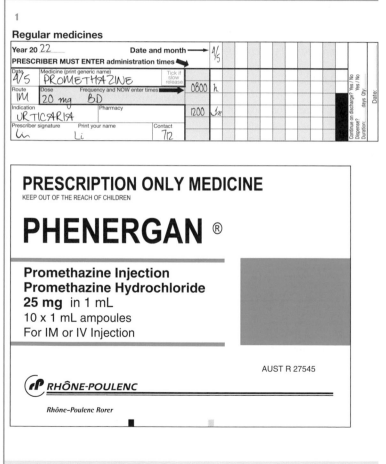

1

Regular medicines

Year 20 22   Date and month → 4/5

PRESCRIBER MUST ENTER administration times ↘

Date 4/5	Medicine (print generic name) PROMETHAZINE	Tick if slow release						
Route IM	Dose 20 mg	Frequency and NOW enter times BD	0800	h.				
Indication URTICARIA		Pharmacy	1200	Jn				
Prescriber signature Ln	Print your name Li	Contact 7l2						

Continue on discharge? Yes / No
Dispense? Yes / No
Duration: ____ days Qty: ____ Date: ____

PRESCRIPTION ONLY MEDICINE
KEEP OUT OF THE REACH OF CHILDREN

PHENERGAN ®

Promethazine Injection
Promethazine Hydrochloride
25 mg in 1 mL
10 x 1 mL ampoules
For IM or IV Injection

AUST R 27545

⟨P⟩ RHÔNE-POULENC

Rhône-Poulenc Rorer

Check your answers in chapter 8.

2

Regular medicines

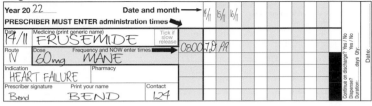

Year 20 22		Date and month →	14/11	15/11	16/11									
PRESCRIBER MUST ENTER administration times ➤														
Date 14/11	Medicine (print generic name) FRUSEMIDE	Tick if slow release	0800	7.9	PA								Continue on discharge? Yes / No	
Route IV	Dose 60mg	Frequency and NOW enter times ➤ MANE											Dispense? Yes / No	Date:
Indication HEART FAILURE		Pharmacy											days Qty: Duration:	
Prescriber signature Bend	Print your name BEND	Contact 124												

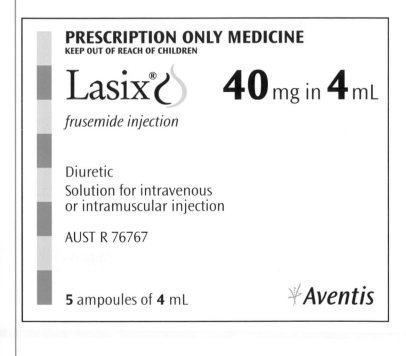

PRESCRIPTION ONLY MEDICINE
KEEP OUT OF REACH OF CHILDREN

Lasix® ⟩ **40** mg in **4** mL

frusemide injection

Diuretic
Solution for intravenous
or intramuscular injection

AUST R 76767

5 ampoules of **4** mL   ⚕*Aventis*

Check your answers in chapter 8.

3

Regular medicines

Year 20 22		Date and month →	¹¹/₁₂											Continue on discharge? Yes / No
First prescriber to print patient name and check label correct:														
Date 11/12	Medicine (print generic name) PROMETHAZINE	Tick if slow release	Date	¹¹/₁₂										Yes / No
Route IM	Dose 12.5 mg Hourly frequency **PRN**	Max PRN dose/24 hrs 3	Time	0630										days Qty:
Indication URTICARIA	Pharmacy		Dose	12.5										Dispenser?
			Route	IM										Duration:
Prescriber signature PK	Print your name KORT	Contact 756	Sign	ℒ										Date:

PRESCRIPTION ONLY MEDICINE
KEEP OUT OF THE REACH OF CHILDREN

PHENERGAN ®

Promethazine Injection
Promethazine Hydrochloride
25 mg in 1 mL
10 x 1 mL ampoules
For IM or IV Injection

AUST R 27545

rP RHÔNE-POULENC

Rhône-Poulenc Rorer

Check your answers in chapter 8.

4

Regular medicines

Year 20 22		Date and month ⟶	3/10	4/10	5/10										
PRESCRIBER MUST ENTER administration times ⟶															

Date 3/10	Medicine (print generic name) FRUSEMIDE		Tick if slow release	0800	η	1/0				Continue on discharge? Yes / No
Route IV	Dose 35 mg	Frequency and NOW enter times BD								Dispense? Yes / No
Indication O EDEMA		Pharmacy		1200	η	73				days Qty.
Prescriber signature Kodg	Print your name KODGI		Contact 891							Duration: _____ Date:

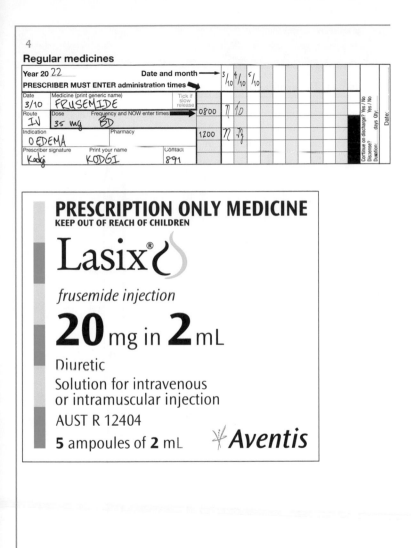

PRESCRIPTION ONLY MEDICINE
KEEP OUT OF REACH OF CHILDREN

Lasix®

frusemide injection

20 mg in **2** mL

Diuretic
Solution for intravenous
or intramuscular injection

AUST R 12404

5 ampoules of **2** mL   ✶ *Aventis*

Check your answers in chapter 8.

9. MEASURING LIQUID VOLUMES FOR INJECTION USING SYRINGES

Exercise 4J *The drawings represent syringes (needles not shown)*

1. For this set of 1 mL syringes, write down the volume (millilitre(s)) of solution
   a. between adjacent graduations
   b. indicated by arrows A, B, C and D.

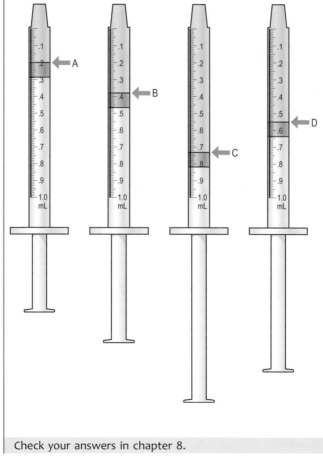

Check your answers in chapter 8.

2. For this set of three syringes, write down the volume (millilitre(s)) of solution
   a. between adjacent graduations
   b. indicated by arrows A, B and C.

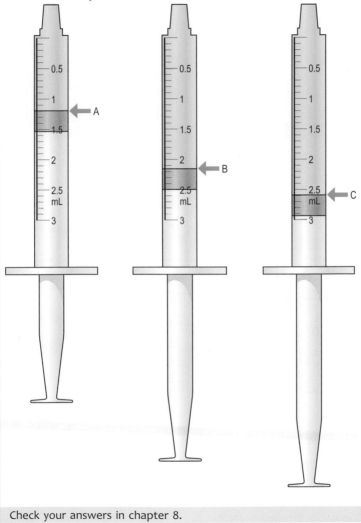

Check your answers in chapter 8.

3. For these syringes, write down the volume (millilitre(s)) of solution
   a. between adjacent graduations
   b. indicated by arrows A, B and C.

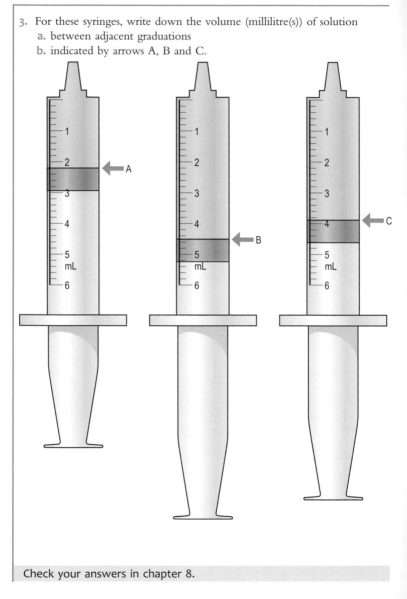

Check your answers in chapter 8.

4. For these 10 mL syringes, write down the volume (millilitre(s)) of solution
   a. between adjacent graduations
   b. indicated by arrows A, B and C.

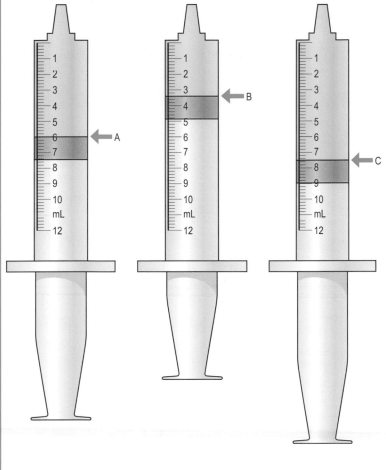

5. These syringes are graduated in *units*, especially for *insulin* injections. Write down the number of units of solution
   a. between adjacent graduations
   b. indicated by arrows A, B, C and D.

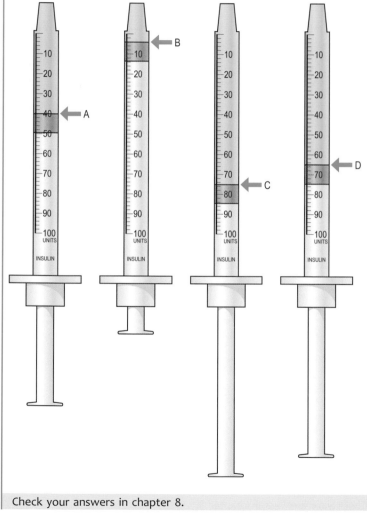

Check your answers in chapter 8.

Dosage calculations for liquid medications

6. For these 50 unit syringes, identify the number of units of solution
   a. between adjacent graduations
   b. indicated by arrows A, B, C and D.

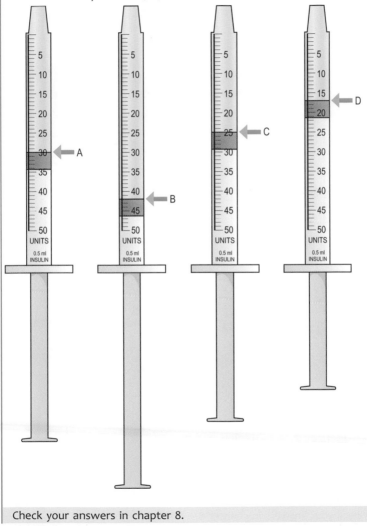

Check your answers in chapter 8.

7. For these 50 unit syringes, note carefully the number of units of solution
   a. between adjacent graduations
   b. indicated by arrows A, B, C and D.

Check your answers in chapter 8.

10. CASE SCENARIO

Chloe is an adolescent with an eating disorder. She is 16 years old and currently weighs 48 kg. Chloe has had several admissions to hospital for anorexia nervosa. Initially, Chloe is prescribed an energy drink to supplement her intake. That is, a compact protein energy drink with meals to deliver 0.84 g of protein per kilogram of body weight each day. The stock available contains 18 g of protein in each 125 mL bottle.

1. Calculate Chloe's daily protein requirement to meet the prescribed dose each day.
2. How many full bottles of the energy drink does Chloe need to consume each day to meet her daily protein requirement?
3. How much liquid will Chloe consume to achieve this daily requirement?

   Chloe drinks 1.5 bottles of the energy drink during her first day on this nutritional regimen.
4. Calculate (in millilitres) the difference between the amount of energy drink needed and what was consumed.

   Chloe's condition continues to decline because she is not consuming enough calories to sustain normal body functions. She is admitted to an adolescent mental health unit. A nasogastric tube is inserted, and a cyclic enteral nutrition regimen was added to supplement Chloe's oral intake. The flow rate was set at 2 mL/min for 24 hrs of continuous enteral feeding.
5. How many millilitres of the enteral nutrition liquid will be administered each day?
6. Convert the answer to litres (L).

   NB: Do not use a trailing zero in the answer because trailing zeros are a source of medication errors when the number is misread.

   In addition to Chloe's cyclic enteral nutrition, the doctor prescribed two other intramuscular supplements. They are cyanocobalamin (B_{12}) 5 mg daily for 5 days and iron polymaltose complex 200 mg second daily until the desired blood haemoglobin level is reached.

7. Calculate the B$_{12}$ daily dose in millilitres if the stock solution is 20 mg/mL.

8. What sized syringe would be best to administer the cyanocobalamin injection?

   The iron polymaltose complex is supplied as 100 mg/2 mL ampoules.

9. Calculate the dose.

10. How many ampoules are required to achieve the correct dose?

    To stabilize Chloe's mood, the prescriber orders a small dose of intramuscular flupentixol decanoate 5 mg. This medication comes in 1 mL ampoules of 20 mg of medication.

11. How much flupentixol decanoate will you give?

    Chloe is on her way to recovery, but before she is discharged, she is given the human papillomavirus (HPV) vaccine. HPV vaccine is in a 0.5 mL mono-dose vial.

12. What syringe will you use to administer this dose?

Dosage calculations for infused medications 5

CHAPTER CONTENTS

1. INTRODUCTION

This chapter deals with the arithmetic of fluid flow rates and drip rates for intravenous (IV) infusion.

The fluid being infused passes from a flask (or similar container) into a giving set (administration set), which has a drip chamber. The giving set may be free-hanging or attached to a volumetric infusion pump.

If the giving set is free-hanging, the nurse needs to calculate the drops per minute to be infused. The nurse can then manipulate the roller clamp on the giving set to ensure the drip rate is correct.

By contrast, if the giving set is connected to an infusion pump, then the nurse needs only to calculate the number of millilitres per hour to be infused and set the pump accordingly.

There may be a holding chamber called a burette between the bag and the giving set. The use of a burette will depend on institution policy and the type of infusion.

Skills covered in this chapter include the following:

- calculating the volume of fluid delivered to a patient over a given time
- infusion pump settings
- rates of flow in millilitres per hour
- rates of flow in drops per minute.

24-hour time will be used in some exercises.

SAFETY MESSAGES

An IV cannula must be inserted to infuse fluid directly into the circulatory system of the body. The condition of the patient is often serious in circumstances where IV fluids and medications are needed. Hence, correctly calculating the rate of the infusion, and closely monitoring the infusion, and the patient response to the infusion is essential. Likewise, special observation of the cannula site is required to ensure that the infused fluid is entering the blood stream and not the interstitial cellular spaces. Smaller amounts of fluid and liquid medications can be infused into arteries, subcutaneously, intrathecally and by intraosseous and epidural routes. Similar and sometimes additional precautions and safety procedures apply to these types of delivery. Similarly, a nutrient fluid infusion, administered through a nasogastric or percutaneous endoscopic gastrostomy tube, must be at the correct rate and assessed for its precise gastrointestinal positioning.

2. WHAT YOU NEED TO KNOW

There are two *main* types of parenteral giving sets in general use — these deliver fluid by drops as a *drop factor* of either 20 or 60 drops/ mL. A drip chamber that delivers 60 drops/mL (or has a *drop factor* of 60 drops/mL) is also known as a microdrip. Another and less common giving set with a drop factor of 15 drops/mL is used (macrodrip) sometimes. Conversely, although either of the two main giving sets can be used for a subcutaneous infusion, it is more common that specialized equipment such as a syringe driver is used. Therefore, the equipment used to administer a fluid infusion will vary depending on the route and indication for fluid therapy. For example, enteral giving sets rarely have drip chambers. Instead, they are designed to connect to the nutrient solution bag and have soft tubing that is massaged by the enteral food pump to deliver a prescribed millilitres per hour dose.

Note: There are several variations of volumetric pumps and accessories. You must know which set to use and in what circumstances.

Important: If in any doubt about the type of giving set or the answer to a calculation, then ask a practice supervisor to check your work.

Refer to prelim page ix for explanations of abbreviations.

3. CALCULATING VOLUME OF AN INFUSION

Example A *A patient is receiving 5% dextrose by IV infusion. The infusion pump is set to deliver 45 mL/hr. Calculate how much fluid the patient will receive in each case.*

How much fluid will the patient receive?

a. **over 2 hrs**   b. **over 3 hrs**   c. **over 7 hrs?**

$$\text{Volume (mL)} = \text{Rate (mL/hr)} \times \text{Time (hrs)}$$

a. 45 mL/hr $\times$ 2 hrs = 90 mL
b. 45 mL/hr $\times$ 3 hrs = 135 mL
c. 45 mL/hr $\times$ 7 hrs = 315 mL

4. CALCULATING TIME FOR AN INFUSION

Example B *A teenager is to receive 750 mL of Hartmann's solution. An infusion pump is set at 60 mL/hr. How long will it take to give the solution?*

$$\text{Time (hrs)} = \frac{\text{Volume (mL)}}{\text{Rate (mL/hr)}}$$

$$= \frac{750 \text{ mL}}{60 \text{mL/hr}}$$

$$= 12\tfrac{1}{2} \text{ hrs} \quad 12 \text{ hrs } 30 \text{ min}$$

$$\text{Simplifying:} \frac{750}{60} = \frac{75}{6} = \frac{25}{2} = 12\tfrac{1}{2}$$

Dosage calculations for infused medications

✏ Exercise 5A

1. An IV cannula has been inserted in a patient. Fluid is being delivered at a rate of 42 mL/hr. How much fluid will the patient receive over **a.** 2 hrs **b.** 8 hrs **c.** 12 hrs?

2. A male patient is receiving Hartmann's solution at a rate of 125 mL/hr. How much solution will he receive over **a.** 3 hrs **b.** 5 hrs **c.** 12 hrs?

3. A girl is to be given 5% dextrose by an infusion pump. If the pump is set at 60 mL/hr, how much 5% dextrose will she receive in **a.** $1\frac{1}{2}$ hrs **b.** $2\frac{1}{2}$ hrs **c.** 12 hrs?

4. A female patient is to receive 500 mL of 0.9% sodium chloride. The infusion rate is adjusted to deliver 25 mL/hr. How long will the 500 mL bag of fluid last?

5. A young man is to be given 1 L of 4% dextrose and $\frac{1}{5}$ normal saline. The infusion pump is set at a rate of 80 mL/hr. What time will it take to give the litre of solution?

6. Half a litre of normal saline with 2 g potassium chloride is to be given to a patient IV. How long will this take if the infusion pump is set at 75 mL/hr?

7. A patient is to receive 100 mL of 0.9% sodium chloride IV. If the infusion pump is set to deliver 150 mL/hr, how long will the infusion take?

8. A male patient is receiving 5% dextrose at a rate of 55 mL/hr. How much fluid will he receive in **a.** 2 hrs **b.** 5 hrs **c.** 11 hrs?

9. A patient is prescribed 500 mL of 0.9% sodium chloride with 10% dextrose. The rate is set at 200 mL/hr. How long will the infusion take?

10. A patient has been prescribed maintenance fluid at a rate of 62 mL/hr. How much fluid will the patient receive over **a.** 6 hrs **b.** 12 hrs **c.** 24 hrs?

11. A patient has been prescribed 300 mL of red cells to be given at a rate of 75 mL/hr. How long will the infusion take?

12. Hartmann's solution of 1L is set at a rate of 84 mL a prescribed. How much will the patient receive in **a.** 4 hrs **b.** 10 hrs **c.** 14 hrs?

Check your answers in chapter 8.

Gatford and Phillips' Drug Calculations

5. CALCULATING RATES OF FLOW IN MILLILITRES PER HOUR (mL/hr) *GIVEN THE TIME IN HOURS*

In order to do this type of calculation, you will need to remember this formula:

$$\text{Rate (mL/hr)} = \frac{\text{Volume (mL)}}{\text{Time (hrs)}}$$

Note: The volume must be in millilitres (mL).

Example *A patient is to receive half a litre of IV fluid over 6 hrs using an infusion pump. At how many millilitres per hour should the pump be set?*

The pump does not have a decimal setting, so calculate the answer to the nearest whole number.

Half a litre = 500 mL

$$\text{Rate (mL/hr)} = \frac{\text{Volume (mL)}}{\text{Time (hrs)}}$$

$$= \frac{500 \text{ mL}}{6 \text{ hrs}}$$

$$= \frac{250}{3} \text{ mL/hr}$$

$$\Rightarrow 83 \text{ mL/hr (to nearest whole number)}$$

$$3\overline{)25^10.^10}$$
$$83.\textcircled{3}$$

Dosage calculations for infused medications

 Exercise 5B *Calculate the required flow rate of a volumetric infusion pump for each of the following infusions.*

Give answers in millilitres per hour to the nearest whole number.

1. One litre of normal saline is to be administered over 8 hrs.

2. A patient is to receive 500 mL of 5% dextrose over 12 hrs.

3. Five hundred millilitres of Hartmann's solution is to be given to a teenager over 7 hrs.

4. Over the next 15 hrs, a female patient is to receive 2 L of 4% dextrose and $\frac{1}{5}$ normal saline.

5. A teenager is to receive 1 L of 0.9% sodium chloride over 6 hrs.

6. A woman is to be given 500 mL of 5% dextrose over 8 hrs.

7. Over a period of 16 hrs, a patient is to receive 1 L of 4% dextrose and 0.18% sodium chloride.

8. A patient is to be given 1 L of normal saline over 24 hrs.

9. Over the next 9 hrs, a patient is to receive half a litre of 4% dextrose and $\frac{1}{5}$ normal saline. At what flow rate should the volumetric infusion pump be set?

10. One litre of Hartmann's solution is to be given over 12 hrs. Calculate the required flow rate for the volumetric infusion pump.

11. One and a half litres of 4% dextrose and 0.18% sodium chloride over 20 hrs are prescribed for a patient. Calculate the required flow rate setting for a volumetric infusion pump.

12. An infusion pump is to be used to administer 1 L of fluid over 11 hrs. At what flow rate should the pump be set?

Check your answers in chapter 8.

6. CALCULATING RATES OF FLOW IN MILLILITRES PER HOUR (mL/hr) *GIVEN THE TIME IN MINUTES*

In order to do this type of calculation, you will need to remember the final formula below:

$$60 \text{ minutes} = 1 \text{ hour}$$

$$60 \text{ min} = 1 \text{ hr}$$

$$\text{Rate (mL/min)} = \frac{\text{Volume (mL)}}{\text{Time (min)}}$$

$$\text{Rate (mL/hr)} = \text{Rate (mL/min)} \times 60$$

$$\therefore \text{Rate (mL/hr)} = \frac{\text{Volume(mL)} \times 60}{\text{Time (min)}}$$

Note: The volume must be in millilitres (mL).

The time must be in minutes (min).

Example *Seventy-five millilitres of fluid in a burette needs to be infused over 20 min. Calculate the flow rate required in millilitres per hour.*

$$\text{Rate (mL/hr)} = \frac{\text{Volume (mL)} \times 60}{\text{Time (min)}}$$

$$= \frac{75 \text{ mL} \times 60}{20 \text{ min}}$$

$$= 225 \text{ mL/hr}$$

Exercise 5C *Each of the following medications has been added to a burette. Calculate the required pump setting in millilitres per hour for the given infusion time. Give each answer to the nearest whole number.*

Medication	Infusion time
1. 40 mL of fluid containing 600 mg of penicillin	20 min
2. 120 mL of fluid containing 500 mg of vancomycin	50 min
3. 100 mL of fluid containing 1 g of flucloxacillin	30 min
4. 50 mL of fluid containing 0.5 g of potassium chloride	30 min
5. 60 mL of fluid containing 75 mg of ranitidine	35 min
6. 80 mL of fluid containing 80 mg of gentamicin	45 min
7. 75 mL of fluid containing 75 mg of gentamicin	40 min
8. 70 mL of fluid containing 1.2 g of penicillin	25 min
9. 80 mL of fluid containing 750 mg of flucloxacillin	30 min
10. 100 mL of fluid containing metronidazole 500 mg	30 min

Check your answers in chapter 8.

7. CALCULATING RATES OF FLOW IN DROPS PER MINUTE (DROPS/MIN)

When a giving set is free-hanging (no pump is being used), the nurse needs to calculate the flow rate in drops/min. This is so that the nurse can set the drip rate accurately by manipulating the roller clamp whilst observing the drip chamber on the giving set.

Note: Before commencing the calculation, always make sure that you know the *drop factor* for the drip chamber of that giving set. The *drop factor* could be 20 drops/mL (delivers fluid at 20 drops/mL), 60 drops/mL (delivers fluid at 60 drops/mL) or 15 drops/mL (delivers fluid at 15 drops/mL).

In order to do this type of calculation, you will need to remember these formulae:

If the time is given in *minutes*, use the following:

$$\text{Rate (drops/min)} = \frac{\text{Volume (mL)} \times \text{Drop factor (drops/mL)}}{\text{Time (min)}}$$

If the time is given in *hours*, use the following:

$$\text{Rate (drops/min)} = \frac{\text{Volume (mL)} \times \text{Drop factor (drops/mL)}}{\text{Time (hrs)} \times 60}$$

Note: The volume must be in millilitres (mL).

Note: Calculating flow rates in drops/min does not apply when an infusion is being delivered by a volumetric pump, because the pump setting regulates the drops as mL/hr.

Example *A patient is prescribed half a litre of 5% dextrose over 4 hrs. The drip chamber in the administration set delivers 20 drops/mL. Calculate the required drip rate in drops/min.*

Give the answer to the nearest whole number.

Note: Half a litre = 500 mL. Time is given in hours.

$$\text{Rate (drops/min)} = \frac{\text{Volume (mL)} \times \text{Drop factor (drops/mL)}}{\text{Time (hrs)} \times 60}$$

$$= \frac{500 \text{ mL} \times 20 \text{ drops/min}}{4 \text{ hrs} \times 60}$$

$$= \frac{500 \times 20 \text{ drops}}{4 \times 60 \text{ min}}$$

$$= \frac{500}{4} \times \frac{1}{3} \text{ drops/min} \left[\text{since } \frac{20}{60} = \frac{1}{3}\right]$$

$$= \frac{125}{3} \text{ drops/min} \left[\text{since } \frac{500}{4} = 125\right]$$

$$\Rightarrow 42 \text{ drops/min}$$

$$3)\overline{125.^20}$$
$$\overline{\quad 41.\textcircled{6}}$$

Note: In this example, the nurse is required to adjust the roller clamp to set the drip rate accurately (drops/min).

Gatford and Phillips' Drug Calculations

✎ **Exercise 5D** *Calculate the required drip rate in drops per minute.*

Give each answer to the nearest whole number.

1. Seven hundred and fifty millilitres of 5% dextrose is to be given over 5 hrs. The IV set delivers 20 drops/mL.

2. An infant is prescribed 150 mL of Hartmann's solution to run over 6 hrs. The microdrip giving set delivers 60 drops/mL.

3. A teenager is to receive 500 mL of 5% dextrose over 8 hrs. The IV set delivers 20 drops/mL.

4. One half litre of dextrose 4% and $\frac{1}{5}$ normal saline is to run over 12 hrs. The administration set delivers 20 drops/mL.

5. Seven hundred and fifty millilitres of normal saline is to be given to a patient over 9 hrs using a giving set which delivers 20 drops/mL.

6. An adult male is to be given half a litre of 0.9% sodium chloride over 5 hrs using an IV set which gives 20 drops/mL.

7. A female patient is to receive $1\frac{1}{2}$ L of fluid over 10 hrs. The giving set delivers 20 drops/mL.

8. A patient is to have the remaining 300 mL of 5% dextrose administered in 50 min. The administration set gives 20 drops/mL.

9. Four hundred millilitres of normal saline is to be infused over 10 hrs using a microdrop giving set. The set delivers 60 drops/mL.

10. A child is prescribed 24 mL/hr of 0.9% sodium chloride. The microdrop giving set delivers 60 drops/mL.

11. An antibiotic has been added to the burette on a giving set. The burette then contains 120 mL of fluid that needs to be delivered in 30 min. The administration set gives 20 drops/mL.

12. A male patient is to have the remaining 50 mL of 5% dextrose infused in 45 min. The administration set gives 20 drops/mL.

Check your answers in chapter 8.

8. CALCULATING RATES OF FLOW FOR BLOOD TRANSFUSIONS (DROPS/MIN)

⚠️ *ALERT!* Blood transfusions are a high-risk procedure. Even though it is rare these days, recipients can have fatal reactions. Every precaution must be taken when calculating the administration rate. Pay attention to the volume of each bag because the volume of every unit of whole blood, packed red blood cells, platelets or plasma can vary. Additionally, the patient must be monitored closely for adverse effects. Adhere to health service policy and protocol.

Example *One unit of packed cells is prescribed to be infused over 2 hrs. The volume of the unit of packed cells is 250 mL. The IV set delivers 20 drops/mL. Calculate the drip rate in drops per minute.*

Give the answer to the nearest whole number.

📝 *Note:* Time is given in hours.

$$\text{Rate (drops/min)} = \frac{\text{Volume (mL)} \times \text{Drop factor (drops/mL)}}{\text{Time (hrs)} \times 60}$$

$$= \frac{250 \text{ mL} \times 20 \text{ drops/mL}}{2 \text{ hrs} \times 60}$$

$$= \frac{250 \times 20 \text{ drops}}{2 \times 60 \text{ min}}$$

$$= \frac{250}{2} \times \frac{1}{3} \text{ drops/min} \left[\text{since } \frac{20}{60} = \frac{1}{3}\right]$$

$$= \frac{125}{3} \text{ drops/min}$$

$$\Rightarrow 42 \text{ drops/min}$$

$$3\overline{)125.^20} $$
$$41.\textcircled{6}$$

📝 *Note:* In this example, the nurse is required to adjust the roller clamp to set the drip rate accurately (drops/min).

Exercise 5E *Calculate the drip rate in drops per minute for each of the following blood transfusions.*

Give each answer to the nearest whole number.

1. An anemic patient is prescribed 1 unit of packed cells over 4 hrs. The unit of packed cells holds 250 mL. The IV set delivers 20 drops/mL.

2. A post–operative adult male is to be given 1 unit of autologous blood in 4 hrs. The unit of autologous blood has a volume of 500 mL. The giving set emits 20 drops/mL.

3. During a transfusion, the doctor prescribes the remaining half unit of packed cells to be administered over 1 hr. A full unit of packed cells is 250 mL. The IV giving set delivers 20 drops/mL.

4. Three hundred millilitres of autologous blood is to be transfused over 2 hrs using an administration set which gives 20 drops/mL.

5. One unit of packed red cells is to be run over 3 hrs. The unit of packed cells contains 350 mL. An IV set which emits 15 drops/mL is to be used.

6. A patient is to be given 1 unit of autologous blood over 3 hrs using a giving set which delivers 15 drops/mL. The unit of blood contains 480 mL.

7. An administration set which emits 15 drops/mL is to be used to give a 480 mL unit of autologous blood over $3\frac{1}{2}$ hrs.

8. A 350 mL unit of packed cells is to be run over $2\frac{1}{2}$ hrs using an IV giving set which delivers 15 drops/mL.

9. Three hundred and fifty millilitres of fresh frozen plasma is to be run over 1 hr using an IV giving set which delivers 15 drops/mL.

10. One unit of packed cells is to be given to a patient over 3 hrs. The giving set delivers 20 drops/mL. Calculate the drip rate in drops per minute if 1 unit of packed cells contains 250 mL.

Check your answers in chapter 8.

9. CALCULATING FINISHING TIMES OF INTRAVENOUS INFUSIONS

⚠ For continuity of fluid therapy, it is essential that nurses be proactive and know when an infusion will finish to ensure that, if needed, follow-up prescriptions are available. Otherwise, there is risk to the patient of interrupted care and inconvenience to the staff who have to arrange another prescription.

Example A *A patient is ordered 1 L of normal saline to be run over $12\frac{1}{2}$ hrs. If the infusion begins at 0800 hrs Monday, calculate the finishing time.*

0800 hrs Monday + 12 hrs 30 min = 2030 hrs Monday

Example B *A patient is to be given 1 L of 5% dextrose over 18 hrs, starting at 0930 hrs Wednesday. Calculate the finishing time.*

0930 hrs Wednesday + 18 hrs 00 min = 2730 hrs

But there are only 24 hrs in a day

2730 hrs − 2400 hrs = 0330 hrs Thursday

Exercise 5F *Calculate the finishing time of each infusion.*

Give each answer in 24-hours time and include the day.

1. *Ordered:* 500 mL normal saline
   Running time: 6 hrs 30 min
   Starting time: 0900 hrs Tuesday

2. *Ordered:* 1 L dextrose 4% and $\frac{1}{5}$ normal saline
   Running time: 13 hrs
   Starting time: Noon Sunday

3. *Ordered:* 1 L of Hartmann's solution
   Running time: 14 hrs
   Starting time: 0730 hrs Friday

4. *Ordered:* 500 mL of dextrose 5%
   Running time: $10\frac{1}{2}$ hrs
   Starting time: 1715 hrs Thursday

5. *Ordered:* 1.2 L of 0.9% sodium chloride
   Running time: $13\frac{1}{2}$ hrs
   Starting time: 1030 hrs Monday

6. *Ordered:* 1.25 L of 4% dextrose and 0.18% sodium chloride
   Running time: 21 hrs
   Starting time: 0900 hrs Saturday

7. *Ordered:* 1 L of Hartmann's solution
   Running time: $11\frac{1}{2}$ hrs
   Starting time: 1300 hrs Wednesday

Check your answers in chapter 8.

10. CALCULATING RUNNING TIMES AND FINISHING TIMES OF INTRAVENOUS INFUSIONS

In order to do this type of calculation, you will need to remember the formulae used in the next two examples.

Example A *At 0730 hrs, a 500 mL bag of 0.9% sodium chloride is set up to run at 80 mL/hr. At what time would the flask have to be replaced?*

$$\text{Running time (hours)} = \frac{\text{Volume (mL)}}{\text{Rate (mL/hr)}}$$

$$= \frac{500 \text{ mL}}{80 \text{ mL/hr}}$$

$$= 6\tfrac{1}{4} \text{ hrs or } 6 \text{ hrs } 15 \text{ min}$$

$$\therefore \text{Finishing time} = 0730 \text{ hrs} + 6 \text{ hrs } 15 \text{ min} = 1345 \text{ hrs}$$

Example B *At 0600 hrs, a 1 L bag of normal saline is set up to run through an infusion pump at 70 mL/hr. After 8 hrs, the flow rate prescribed is to be increased to 80 mL/hr. By what time would the flask have to be replaced?*

i. Volume (mL) = Rate (mL/hr) × Time (hrs)

= 70 mL/hr × 8 hrs = 560 mL

$= 5\frac{1}{2}$ hrs or 5 hrs 30 min

ii. One litre = 1000 mL

∴ Volume remaining = 1000 mL − 560 mL = 440 mL

iii. Running time (hours) $= \dfrac{\text{Volume (mL)}}{\text{Rate (mL/hr)}}$

$= \dfrac{440 \text{ mL}}{80 \text{ mL/hr}}$

$= 5\frac{1}{2}$ hrs or 5 hrs 30 min

iv. Total running time $= 8 \text{ hrs} + 5\frac{1}{2} \text{ hrs} = 13\frac{1}{2}$ hrs or 13 hrs 30 min

v. ∴ Finishing time = 0600 hrs + 13 hrs 30 min = 1930 hrs

Dosage calculations for infused medications

Exercise 5G

1. A patient has *two* IV lines. One line is being infused at 45 mL/hr; the other at 30 mL/hr. What volume of fluid would this patient receive in a 24-hour period?

2. At 0800 hrs, 1 L of 4% dextrose and 0.18% sodium chloride are set up to run at 75 mL/hr. At what time would the flask be finished?

3. At 2100 hrs on a Monday, 1 L of 5% dextrose is set up to run at 50 mL/hr. When will the flask be finished?

4. One litre of Hartmann's solution is to be given by IV. For the first 6 hrs, the solution is delivered at 85 mL/hr, then the rate is prescribed to be reduced to 70 mL/hr. Find the total time taken to give the full volume.

5. A patient is to receive half a litre of 5% dextrose by IV. A flask is set up at 0800 hrs running at 60 mL/hr. After 5 hrs, the rate is prescribed to be increased to 80 mL/hr. At what time will the IV be completed?

6. At 0430 hrs, an infusion pump is set to deliver 1.5 L of fluid at a rate of 90 mL/hr. After 10 hrs, the pump is reset to 75 mL/hr. Calculate the finishing time.

7. A 1 L IV flask of 0.9% sodium chloride has been infused for 6 hrs at a rate of 75 mL/hr. The doctor prescribes the remaining volume to be run through in the next 5 hrs. Calculate the new flow rate.

8. A patient is to receive 1 L of 4% dextrose and 0.18% sodium chloride. For the first $3\frac{1}{2}$ hrs, the fluid is delivered at 160 mL/hr. A specialist then prescribes that the rate be slowed so that the remaining fluid will run over the next 8 hrs. Calculate the required flow rate.

9. A patient is receiving fluid from *two* IV lines. One line is running at 65 mL/hr; the other at 70 mL/hr. What volume of fluid would the patient receive by IV over 12 hrs?

10. At 0700 hrs, half a litre of 5% dextrose is set up to run at 40 mL/hr. At what time will the flask be finished?

Check your answers in chapter 8.

11. One litre of 5% dextrose is to be given by IV. The solution is to run at 75 mL/hr for the first 6 hrs, then the rate is to be reduced to 50 mL/hr. Calculate the *total* time required to give the full volume.

12. At 0300 hrs, 2 L of 0.9% sodium chloride is set up to be delivered through an infusion pump at 85 mL/hr. After 8 hrs, the prescribed rate is increased to 120 mL/hr. Calculate the finishing time.

Check your answers in chapter 8.

11. CALCULATING STOCK CONCENTRATION AND ADMINISTRATION OF DOSAGES

⚠️ *Important:* There are times when the nurse needs to add a medication to a diluent solution to make up an amount of medication for infusion. Therefore, understanding the process for calculating the stock concentration is essential for accurate administration of medication dosages. Additionally, you must know the displacement value of the medication being added to the diluent. That is, the measure of the medication that occupies space in the diluent container.

⚙️ **In order to do this type of calculation, you will need to remember the following four formulae:**

1. To calculate the concentration of a stock solution, use the following:

$$\text{Concentration of stock (mg/mL)} = \frac{\text{Stock strength (mg)}}{\text{Volume of stock solution (mL)}}$$

2. To calculate the amount of medication contained in a given volume, use the following:

$$\text{Dosage (mg)} = \text{Volume (mL)} \times \text{Concentration of stock (mg/mL)}$$

3. To calculate the amount of medication received per hour, use the following:

$$\text{hourly dosage (mg/hr)} = \text{Rate (mL/hr)} \times \text{Concentration of stock (mg/mL)}$$

4. To calculate the rate in millilitres per hour, use the following:

$$\text{Rate (mL/hr)} = \frac{\text{hourly dosage (mg/hr)}}{\text{Concentration of stock (mg/mL)}}$$

Gatford and Phillips' Drug Calculations

Example A *A young post-operative patient's IV analgesic prescription is for pethidine 300 mg in 500 mL of normal saline. The solution is prescribed to run between 10 and 40 mL/hr, depending on the nurse's assessment of pain.*

a. **Calculate the concentration of the pethidine/saline solution.**
b. **How many milligrams of pethidine will the patient receive each hour if the infusion is run at 25 mL/hr?**
c. **At what rate (in mL/hr) should the nurse set the pump to administer the pethidine at 8 mg/hr? Give answer to nearest whole number.**

a. Concentration $= \dfrac{300 \text{ mg}}{500 \text{ mL}} = \dfrac{3}{5}$ mg/mL or 0.6 mg/mL

b. Hourly dosage $= 25 \text{ mL/hr} \times 0.6 \text{ mg/mL} = 15 \text{ mg/mL}$

c. Rate $= \dfrac{8 \text{ mg/hr}}{0.6 \text{ mg/mL}} = \dfrac{80}{6}$ mL/hr $= 13.3 \Rightarrow 13$ mL/hr

$6)8^20.^20$
$13.\circled{3}$

Example B *A post-operative female patient has a patient-controlled analgesia (PCA) infusion. The flask contains morphine 50 mg in 100 mL of normal saline. The PCA has been set, as per doctor's prescription, so that when the patient presses the button she receives a bolus dose of 1 mL.*

a. **Calculate the concentration of the morphine/saline solution.**
b. **How much morphine does the bolus dose contain?**

a. Concentration $= \dfrac{50 \text{ mg}}{100 \text{ mL}} = \dfrac{1}{2}$ mg/mL $= 0.5$ mg/mL

b. Dosage (mg) = Volume (mL) × Concentration of stock (mg/mL)

∴ Dosage $= 1 \text{ mL} \times 0.5 \text{ mg/mL} = 0.5$ mg

Exercise 5H

1. A young post-operative patient is prescribed pethidine 350 mg in 500 mL of normal saline. The solution is prescribed to infuse between 10 and 40 mL/hr, depending on the nurse's assessment of pain.
   a. What is the concentration (milligrams per millilitre) of the pethidine/saline solution?
   b. How many milligrams of pethidine will the patient receive hourly if the infusion is run at
      i. 10 mL/hr
      ii. 15 mL/hr
      iii. 25 mL/hr
      iv. 40 mL/hr?

   c. At what rate (millilitres per hour) should the pump be set to deliver the pethidine at
      i. 9 mg/hr
      ii. 12 mg/hr
      iii. 20 mg/hr
      iv. 25 mg/hr?

   [Give each answer to nearest whole number.]

2. An adult male patient is prescribed morphine 50 mg in 500 mL of normal saline. The solution is to be infused at 10–40 mL/hr using a volumetric infusion pump.
   a. Calculate the concentration (milligrams per millilitre) of the morphine/saline solution.
   b. How many milligrams of morphine will the patient receive per hour if the pump is set at
      i. 10 mL/hr
      ii. 15 mL/hr
      iii. 20 mL/hr
      iv. 40 mL/hr?

   c. At what rate (millilitres per hour) should the pump be set to deliver the morphine at
      i. 1.5 mg/hr
      ii. 2.5 mg/hr
      iii. 3 mg/hr
      iv. 3.5 mg/hr?

Check your answers in chapter 8.

3. A post-operative patient has a PCA infusion running via a syringe pump. The syringe contains fentanyl 300 micrograms in 30 mL of 0.9% sodium chloride. The PCA has been set, in accordance with doctor's prescription, so that when the button is pressed the patient receives a bolus dose of 1 mL.
   a. What is the concentration (microgram per millilitre) of the solution in the syringe?
   b. How much fentanyl is in each bolus dose?
   c. If the patient has six bolus doses within an hour, how much fentanyl has the patient received in that hour?

4. A post-operative patient is prescribed morphine 25 mg in 50 mL of normal saline via an infusion pump.
   a. Calculate the concentration (milligrams per millilitre) of the morphine/saline solution.
   b. How many milligrams of morphine will the patient receive hourly if the pump is set at 5 mL/hr?
   c. At what rate (millilitres per hour) should the pump be set to deliver morphine at 3.5 mg/hr?

5. A post-operative patient is receiving a PCA infusion of fentanyl 250 micrograms in 25 mL of normal saline via a syringe pump. The PCA is set to give a bolus dose of 1 mL each time the button is pressed.
   a. What is the concentration (microgram per millilitre) of the fentanyl/saline solution?
   b. How much fentanyl is in each bolus dose?
   c. If the patient has five bolus doses between 1400 hrs and 1500 hrs on a Sunday, how much fentanyl has the patient received in that hour?

Check your answers in chapter 8.

12. CALCULATING KILOJOULES OF ENERGY

⚠ *Important:* Calculating the number of kilojoules a patient receives from an IV infusion is not something that a nurse does regularly. However, in certain patient situations, it is beneficial to be aware of the number of kilojoules the patient is receiving from the infusion. Similarly, if the patient is receiving total parenteral nutrition in the form of fluid therapy, then calculating the kilojoules received is part of the clinical management.

🔋 *Note:* Dextrose and glucose are carbohydrates. The given percentage of dextrose (or glucose) is equal to the number of grams of dextrose (or glucose) per 100 mL of solution.

For example

> 5% dextrose = 5 g of dextrose per 100 mL of solution
> 10% dextrose = 10 g of dextrose per 100 mL of solution
> 25% dextrose = 25 g of dextrose per 100 mL of solution
> 50% dextrose = 50 g of dextrose per 100 mL of solution

Example *One gram of dextrose provides 16 kJ of energy. How many kilojoules does a patient receive from an infusion of $1\frac{1}{2}$ L of 10% dextrose?*

10% dextrose = 10 g of dextrose per 100 mL of solution

$$= \frac{10 \text{ g}}{100 \text{ mL}}$$

$$1\frac{1}{2} \text{ L} = 1500 \text{ mL}$$

Weight of dextrose (g) = Volume of infusion (mL)

$$\times \text{ strength of solution (g/100 mL)}$$

$$= 1500 \text{ mL} \times \frac{10 \text{ g}}{100 \text{ mL}}$$

$$= \frac{1500 \text{ mL}}{1} \times \frac{10 \text{ g}}{100 \text{ mL}}$$

$$= 15 \times 10 \text{ g} \quad (1500 \text{ mL} \div 100 \text{ mL} = 15)$$

$$= 150 \text{ g}$$

Energy supplied = 150 g × 16 kJ/g

$$= 2400 \text{ kJ}$$

Exercise 5I *One gram of carbohydrate provides 16 kJ of energy. Dextrose and glucose are carbohydrates. Calculate how many kilojoules will be received by a patient during each of the following infusions.*

1. 1 L of 5% dextrose

2. $2\frac{1}{2}$ L of 5% dextrose

3. 1 L of 10% dextrose

4. 500 mL of 25% dextrose

5. 2 L of normal saline
    [Normal saline is a 0.9% solution of salt in water.]

6. 750 mL of 4% dextrose and $\frac{1}{5}$ normal saline

7. $1\frac{1}{2}$ L of Hartmann's solution
    [Hartmann's solution contains sodium lactate, sodium chloride, potassium chloride and calcium chloride.]

8. A patient with diabetes is found unconscious and presumed to be hypo-glycaemic. Fifty millilitres of 50% glucose is given to the patient. How many kilojoules of energy are administered in the 50 mL dose?

Check your answers in chapter 8.

13. CASE SCENARIO

Robyn is a 45-year-old female patient in the surgical ward. She has undergone a laparoscopic cholecystectomy for removal of an inflamed gall bladder containing several stones. To manage the acute post-operative pain, the anaesthetic treating team prescribed a continuous IV infusion regimen using fentanyl at a rate of 0.35 microgram/kg/hr for the first 24 hrs.

Robyn weighs 79 kg.

1. Calculate the dose of fentanyl (in micrograms) for adding to the infusion fluid for the first 24-hour period of the infusion.
2. Calculate the dose of fentanyl (in micrograms) to be administered each hour.

Fentanyl is available in an ampoule containing 100 micrograms in 2 mL.

3. Calculate the amount (in millilitres) of the 100 microgram in 2 mL fentanyl stock solution to be added to the IV diluent fluid.

Fentanyl is also available in an ampoule containing 500 micrograms in 10 mL.

4. Calculate the amount (in millilitres) of the 500 microgram in 10 mL fentanyl stock solution you would add to the IV diluent fluid if you were using it.
5. Critical thinking question: Which of the stock solutions is best to use in this case, and why?

The fentanyl is diluted in a 0.9% sodium chloride solution for IV infusion over the 24 hrs. The 0.9% saline solution is supplied as a 100 mL bag.

6. How much of the infusion fluid will you discard to make up to 100 mL after the medication is added?

The infusion is set up, and the rate needs to be set.

7. Calculate the infusion rate required (in millilitres per hour) to deliver the prescribed hourly dose.

Fentanyl is an opioid medication that suppresses the central nervous system. Therefore, close monitoring of Robyn's level of consciousness is essential for safe administration of this medication.

Sedation score

- 0 — wide awake
- 1 — easy to rouse
- 2 — easy to rouse, but cannot stay awake
- 3 — difficult to rouse.

You should aim to keep the sedation score <2 because a score of 2 represents early respiratory depression (Australian Medicines Handbook, 2020, https://amhonline-amh-net-au).

8. Critical thinking question: What would be your response if Robyn's sedation score was 2?

Robyn's pain diminishes after the first 24 hrs post-operatively. The continuous infusion of fentanyl is now not required. The treating medical team determine that IV PCA is more appropriate for moderate pain.

They prescribe a bolus dose of 20 micrograms of fentanyl for each time Robyn initiates the PCA button. The medication is prepared as 1000 micrograms of fentanyl in 100 mL of 0.9% sodium chloride solution — the PCA machine locks for 5 min after each press of the button.

9. How many times can Robyn press the button in each hour?
10. How much medication (in micrograms) will Robyn receive in 1 hr if she presses the button every 5 min?

Please refer to your local protocols to check whether the dose in question 10 is safe. If it is not, then reflect on your action as the responsible nurse in this scenario.

Robyn's blood results reveal that she is dehydrated and has a low potassium.

To correct dehydration and hypokalaemia the treating team order supplementary fluids: The regimen is a primary infusion of sodium chloride 0.9% 1 L eight hourly for 48 hrs with a secondary sideline of pre-mixed 100 mL of 0.9% normal saline and 10 mmoL of potassium at a rate of 2 mmol/hr for 24 hrs.

11. Calculate the drip rate of the primary 0.9% normal saline if it is administered by a giving set that delivers 20 drops/mL.
12. Critical thinking question: Note that IV potassium must be closely monitored and solutions with concentrations higher than 30 mmol/1000 mL must be administered using an infusion pump. Why?

6 | Paediatric dosages

CHAPTER CONTENTS

1. INTRODUCTION

In this chapter, dosages of medications for children will be considered. The exercises focus on the arithmetic of oral medications and injections, *specifically for children*. Intravenous (IV) infusion calculations have been covered in Chapter 5.

By the end of this chapter, you should be able to:

* calculate drug doses related to both body weight and body surface area (BSA).

 SAFETY MESSAGES

Great care must be taken when administering medication to children. *The smallest error is potentially life threatening.*

If there is **any** doubt about the answer to a medication calculation, then ask a supervisor to check your work. Also, check local policy as some health services require two checkers for drug administration in children.

2. WHAT YOU NEED TO KNOW

Children grow at different rates.

There are wide variations in the actual weight of a child of a given age compared to the average weight for a child of that age. For example, those caring for children may encounter a preterm baby weighing only a few hundred grams, as well as an adolescent who may weigh as much as an adult patient. Consequently, dosages are usually calculated according to body weight. In more complex situations, dosages are based on BSA, for example, in chemotherapy.

BSA can be determined using the body weight and height of a child, which can be determined using a commercially accepted chart known as a nomogram (see Section 10). When dealing with an infant (a child aged less than 1 year), body weight and *length* are used.

BSA determines the loss of fluid from the body by evaporation. This fluid loss is critical in the case of some medications, and this is when the BSA is used in a calculation, rather than weight.

The prescription should specify whether to use weight or BSA.

⚠ *Important*: If in **any** doubt about the answer to a calculation, then ask a supervisor to check your work.

Refer to prelim page ix for explanations of abbreviations.

3. CALCULATING A SINGLE DOSE BASED ON BODY WEIGHT

Calculating the size of a single dose is based on the recommended dosage (in milligrams (mg) per kilogram (kg) per day (mg/kg/day)) and a child's weight. The nurse is not usually required to do this calculation. However, it is important that you understand how a single dose prescription is determined.

Note: There is no particular formula required for these calculations.

Example A *A young girl is to be given amoxicillin. The recommended dosage is 30 mg/kg 12 hrly. The girl's weight is 18 kg. How much amoxicillin should she receive in every 12 hrs?*

$$30 \text{ mg/kg} \times 18 \text{ kg} = 540 \text{ mg}$$

Example B *A child is prescribed erythromycin. The recommended dosage is 40 mg/kg/day, in 4 divided doses daily. If the child's weight is 15 kg, calculate the size of a single dose.*

$$15 \text{ kg} \times 40 \text{ mg/kg/day} = 600 \text{ mg/day}$$

Then,

$$600 \text{ mg} \div 4 \text{ doses} = 150 \text{ mg/dose}$$

Exercises 6A

Given each child's weight, calculate the amount of medication to be given 12 hrly.
1. Trimethoprim, 4 mg/kg, 12 hrly, weight 7 kg
2. Phenytoin, 3 mg/kg, 12 hrly, weight 33 kg
3. Spironolactone, 25 mg/kg, 12 hrly, weight 27 kg

Calculate the size of a single dose for a child weighing 12 kg.
4. Erythromycin, 40 mg/kg/day, 4 doses per day
5. Penicillin V, 50 mg/kg/day, 4 doses per day
6. Cefalexin, 30 mg/kg/day, 4 doses per day

Calculate the size of a single dose for a child weighing 20 kg.
7. Cloxacillin, 50 mg/kg/day, 4 doses per day
8. Chloramphenicol, 40 mg/kg/day, 4 doses per day
9. Amoxicillin, 45 mg/kg/day, 4 doses per day

Calculate the size of a single dose for a child weighing 36 kg.
10. Flucloxacillin, 100 mg/kg/day, 4 doses per day
11. Capreomycin sulphate, 20 mg/kg/day, 3 doses per day
12. Cephalothin, 60 mg/kg/day, 4 doses per day

Check your answers in Chapter 8.

4. ESTIMATING VOLUMES FOR INJECTION IN PAEDIATRIC PATIENTS

Medication dosage calculation errors are a common risk in paediatric settings due to the need for more complex dosage calculations. For example, paediatric dosage calculations are often based on individual patient weight, age or BSA as well as the condition being treated. When only a small fraction of the adult dose is required, there can be a higher likelihood of errors, such as a 10-fold or greater dosing due to miscalculation or misplacement of the decimal point.

For these reasons, the concept of estimation of drug doses becomes useful. The estimation concept encourages the administrator to estimate whether the volume of the dose is accurate. If a calculated drug dose does not make sense because it seems to be too large in volume, then it needs to be re-calculated. Thus, estimation will give an indication of whether a drug is less than, equal to or more than the given volume, for example:

Example *A girl is to be given 150 micrograms of digoxin intravenously. Ampoules contain digoxin 0.5 mg in 2 mL. Is the volume to be drawn up for injection equal to 2 mL, less than 2 mL or more than 2 mL?*

The stock ampoule contains 0.5 mg of digoxin
0.5 mg = 500 micrograms
The volume of ampoule = 2 mL
150 micrograms (prescribed) is *less than* 500 micrograms (stock)
Therefore, the volume to be drawn up is *less than* 2 mL

Exercises 6B *Choose the correct answer to each problem. The answer will be equal to, less than or more than the volume of the stock ampoule or vial.*

1. *Prescribed:* pethidine 30 mg
   Stock: pethidine 50 mg in 1 mL
   Is the volume to be drawn up equal to 1 mL, less than 1 mL or more than 1 mL?

2. *Prescribed:* capreomycin sulphate 200 mg
   Stock: capreomycin sulphate 1 g in 5 mL
   Is the volume to be drawn up equal to 5 mL, less than 5 mL or more than 5 mL?

3. *Prescribed:* gentamicin 25 mg
   Stock: gentamicin 20 mg/2 mL
   Is the volume to be drawn up equal to 2 mL, less than 2 mL or more than 2 mL?

4. *Prescribed:* naloxone 20 micrograms
   Stock: naloxone 0.02 mg/mL
   Is the volume to be drawn up equal to 1 mL, less than 1 mL or more than 1 mL?

5. *Prescribed:* atropine 0.5 mg
   Stock: atropine 0.2 mg in 1 mL
   Is the volume to be drawn up equal to 1 mL, less than 1 mL or more than 1 mL?

6. *Prescribed:* flucloxacillin 350 mg
   Stock: flucloxacillin 1 g in 3 mL
   Is the volume to be drawn up equal to 3 mL, less than 3 mL or more than 3 mL?

7. *Prescribed:* gentamicin 45 mg
   Stock: gentamicin 60 mg/1.5 mL
   Is the volume to be drawn up equal to 1.5 mL, less than 1.5 mL or more than 1.5 mL?

Check your answers in Chapter 8.

Paediatric dosages

8. *Prescribed:* aciclovir 120 mg
   Stock: aciclovir 250 mg/10 mL
   Is the volume to be drawn up equal to 10 mL, less than 10 mL or more than 10 mL?

9. *Prescribed:* paracetamol IV 150 mg
   Stock: 100 mg/10 mL
   Is the volume to be drawn up equal to 10 mL, less than 10 mL or more than 10 mL?

10. *Prescribed:* diclofenac sodium 25 mg
    Stock: 25 mg/mL
    Is the volume to be drawn up equal to 1 mL, less than 1 mL or more than 1 mL?

11. *Prescribed:* metronidazole 400 mg
    Stock: 500 mg/100 mL
    Is the volume to be drawn up equal to 100 mL, less than 100 mL or more than 100 mL?

12. *Prescribed:* midazolam 25 mg
    Stock: 50 mg/10 mL
    Is the volume required to be drawn up equal to 10 mL, less than 10 mL or more than 10 mL?

Check your answers in Chapter 8.

5. CALCULATING VOLUMES FOR INJECTION IN PAEDIATRIC PATIENTS

Example A *A boy is prescribed pethidine 35 mg, intramuscular (IM) at 0800 hrs. Stock ampoules contain 50 mg in 1 mL. What volume must be drawn up for injection?*

$$\text{Volume required} = \frac{\text{Strength required}}{\text{Stock strength}} \times [\text{Volume of stock solution}]$$

The formula can be abbreviated to the following:

$$VR = \frac{SR}{SS} \times VS$$

$$= \frac{35 \text{ mg}}{50 \text{ mg}} \times 1 \text{ mL}$$

$$= \frac{35}{50} \text{ mL} = \frac{7}{10} \text{ mL}$$

$$= 0.7 \text{ mL}$$

Example B *A child is prescribed digoxin 40 micrograms, IV. Paediatric ampoules contain 50 micrograms/2 mL. Calculate the amount to be drawn up in a syringe.*

$$\text{Volume required} = \frac{\text{Strength required}}{\text{Stock strength}} \times [\text{Volume of stock solution}]$$

$$VR = \frac{SR}{SS} \times VS$$

$$= \frac{40 \text{ micrograms}}{50 \text{ micrograms}} \times 2 \text{ mL}$$

$$= \frac{40}{50} \times \frac{2}{1} \text{ mL}$$

$$= \frac{80}{50} \text{ mL}$$

$$= \frac{8}{5} \text{ mL}$$

$$= 1.6 \text{ mL}$$

If you are having difficulty simplifying the fractions in these examples, then refer to Review exercises 2H and 2I in Chapter 2.

Exercises 6C *For each of these paediatric dosages, calculate the volume to be drawn up in a syringe for injection.*

Prescribed	Stock
1. Metoclopramide 4 mg	10 mg in 2 mL
2. Atropine 0.3 mg	0.4 mg in 1 mL
3. Digoxin 125 micrograms	0.5 mg/2 mL
4. Digoxin 18 micrograms	50 micrograms in 2 mL
5. Cephalothin 120 mg	500 mg in 2 mL
6. Cephalothin 300 mg	500 mg in 2 mL
7. Flucloxacillin 400 mg	1 g in 3 mL
8. Flucloxacillin 100 mg	1 g in 3 mL
9. Phenobarbital 50 mg	200 mg/mL
10. Aminophylline 180 mg	250 mg in 10 mL
11. Morphine 6.5 mg	10 mg in 1 mL
12. Gentamicin 15 mg	20 mg/2 mL
13. Gentamicin 40 mg	60 mg/1.5 mL
14. Morphine 8 mg	10 mg/mL
15. Furosemide (frusemide) 4.5 mg	20 mg in 2 mL
16. Omnopon 16 mg	20 mg/mL

 Important

- Always check that each answer makes sense.
- Should the volume you calculated be equal to, or less than or more than the volume of the stock ampoule?

Check your answers in Chapter 8.

6. CALCULATING PAEDIATRIC DOSAGES FOR ORAL MEDICATIONS IN LIQUID FORM

Children are frequently prescribed oral medication in liquid form. Liquid medication allows a greater range of specific dosages compared to solid form (tablets and capsules). This is especially relevant for children as there is a great range of weights for a child of a given age. Generally, a child finds a liquid medication easier to take than a tablet or capsule. The liquid medication may be a syrup, an elixir, a solution or a suspension.

⚠ *Important:* Suspensions must be shaken thoroughly before measuring the volume to ensure that all of the medicine particles, which may settle on the bottom, are evenly dispersed to ensure the patient receives the full dose of medication and not just liquid preparation.

Example A *A child is prescribed 80 mg of paracetamol elixir. Stock on hand is 100 mg in 5 mL. Calculate the volume to be given.*

$$\text{Volume required} = \frac{\text{Strength required}}{\text{Stock strength}} \times [\text{Volume of stock solution}]$$

The formula can be abbreviated to the following:

$$VR = \frac{SR}{SS} \times VS$$

$$= \frac{80 \text{ mg}}{100 \text{ mg}} \times 5 \text{ mL}$$

$$= \frac{80}{100} \times \frac{5}{1} \text{ mL}$$

$$= \frac{4}{5} \times \frac{5}{1} \text{ mL} \text{ [The 5s cancel out]}$$

$$= 4 \text{ mL}$$

Example B *A child is to be given 175 micrograms of digoxin, orally. The paediatric mixture contains 50 micrograms/mL. Calculate the required volume.*

$$\text{Volume required} = \frac{\text{Strength required}}{\text{Stock strength}} \times [\text{Volume of stock solution}]$$

The formula can be abbreviated to the following:

$$VR = \frac{SR}{SS} \times VS$$

$$= \frac{175 \text{ micrograms}}{50 \text{ micrograms}} \times 1 \text{ mL}$$

$$= \frac{175}{50} \text{ mL}$$

$$= \frac{35}{10} \text{ mL}$$

$$= \frac{7}{2} \text{ mL}$$

$$= 3.5 \text{ mL}$$

Exercises 6D *Calculate the volume to be given orally for these paediatric dosages.*

Prescribed	Stock
1. 70 mg of paracetamol elixir	100 mg/5 mL
2. 300 mg of paracetamol elixir	120 mg/5 mL
3. 12.5 mg of promethazine elixir	5 mg/5 mL
4. 70 mg of theophylline syrup	50 mg/5 mL
5. 125 micrograms of digoxin elixir	50 micrograms/mL
6. 24 mg of phenytoin suspension	30 mg/5 mL
7. 200 mg of penicillin suspension	125 mg/5 mL
8. 350 mg of penicillin suspension	125 mg/5 mL
9. 60 mg of theophylline syrup	80 mg/15 mL
10. 225 mg of amoxicillin syrup	1 g/10 mL
11. 1.5 mg of clonazepam syrup	2.5 mg/mL
12. 50 mg of amoxicillin syrup	1 g/10 mL
13. 100 mg of flucloxacillin syrup	125 mg/5 mL
14. 180 mg of flucloxacillin syrup	150 mg/5 mL
15. 4 mg of chlorphenamine suspension	2 mg/5 mL
16. 300 mg of ibuprofen suspension	100 mg/5 mL

Check your answers in Chapter 8.

7. CALCULATING PAEDIATRIC DOSAGES OF POWDER-FORM MEDICATIONS FOR INJECTION

Some medications are supplied in vials containing the medication in powder form. The powder must be mixed with a diluent such as water for injection (WFI) before administration. When a known volume of WFI is mixed with the vial of powder, the resulting solution has a volume greater than the volume of the WFI. The concentration of the solution (milligrams per millilitres) depends upon the volume of WFI used. Some medication labels show the various amounts of WFI to be added to the vial to yield given concentrations of solutions. This also gives consideration to the displacement value of the powder.

⚠️ *Important:* Displacement values in powder–form medications should be considered or stated when re constituting the medication. Ignoring displacement measures could result in under-dosing of children.

For example, a medicine in powder form needs to be re-constituted to 10 mL. If the powdered medication in the vial equates to 0.5 mL, then the WFI should be 9.5 mL to give a total volume of 10 mL as indicated. If the administrator was to add 10 mL ignoring the displacement value, then the final volume would be greater than 10 mL (e.g., 10.5 mL). A solution greater than the volume required would subsequently dilute the concentration and dilute the dose.

8. THE VOLUME OF WATER FOR INJECTION AND CONCENTRATION OF A SOLUTION

Below is an example of a WFI table. The amoxicillin in the vial is in powder form.

AMOXICILLIN 500 mg IV VIAL

For a concentration of	100	125	200	250	mg/mL
Add	4.6	3.6	2.1	1.6	mL of WFI

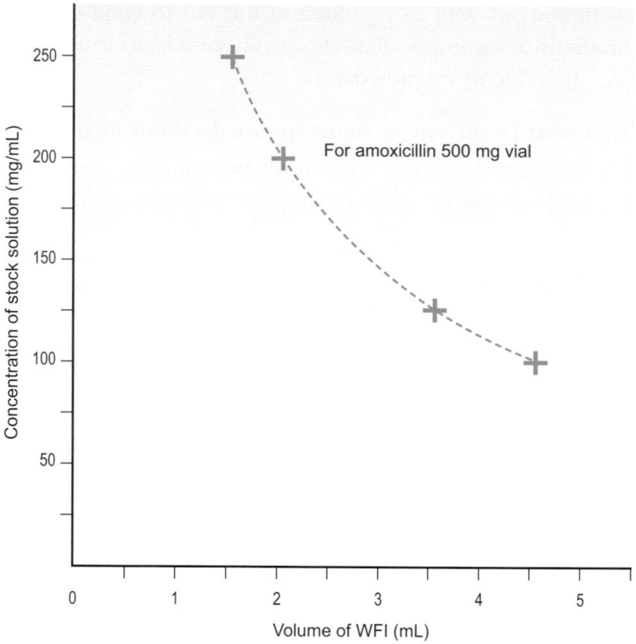

Figure 6.1 The graph illustrates the relationship between concentration of a stock solution and volume of water for injection *(WFI)*.

The table and the graph show how the concentration of a stock solution depends on the volume of WFI mixed with the vial of powder. The bigger the volume of WFI, the lower the concentration of the stock solution.

Example *Stock vial: benzylpenicillin 600 mg.*

For a concentration of:	150	200	300	mg/mL
Add:	3.6	2.6	1.6	mL of WFI

A 12 kg child is prescribed 270 mg of benzylpenicillin, 8-hrly, IV. How much solution should be drawn up for injection if the concentration, after dilution with WFI, is each of the following

a. **150 mg/mL**   b. **200 mg/mL**   c. **300 mg/mL?**

$$\text{Volume required} = \frac{\text{Strength required}}{\text{Stock strength}} \times [\text{Volume of stock solution}]$$

a. Volume required $= \dfrac{270 \text{ mg}}{150 \text{ mg}} \times 1 \text{ mL}$

$= \dfrac{9}{5} \text{ mL}$

$= 1.8 \text{ mL}$

$5\overline{)9.^40}$
$\qquad 1.8$

b. Volume required $= \dfrac{270 \text{ mg}}{200 \text{ mg}} \times 1 \text{ mL}$

$= \dfrac{27}{20} \text{ mL}$

$= 1.35 \text{ mL}$

$= 1.4 \text{ mL (correct to 1 d.p.)}$

$10\overline{)27.0}$
$2\overline{)2.7^10}$
$\qquad 1.35$

c. Volume required $= \dfrac{270 \text{ mg}}{300 \text{ mg}} \times 1 \text{ mL}$

$= \dfrac{9}{10} \text{ mL}$

$= 0.9 \text{ mL}$

⚠ **Exercise 6E** *Give answers greater than 1 mL correct to one decimal place and answers less than 1 mL correct to two decimal places.*

1. An 8 kg child is prescribed 180 mg of benzylpenicillin, IV. How much solution should be drawn up for injection for the following concentrations after dilution with WFI (see benzylpenicillin table on page 161)
   a. 150 mg/mL   b. 200 mg/mL   c. 300 mg/mL?

2. *Prescription:* amoxicillin 150 mg IV
   What volume of solution would need to be drawn up for injection for the following concentrations after dilution with WFI (see amoxicillin table on page 160)
   a. 100 mg/mL   b. 125 mg/mL   c. 200 mg/mL   d. 250 mg/mL?

3. *The label on vial:* Ampicillin 500 mg multiple-dose vial
   Re-constitution: Add 1.8 mL of WFI to yield 250 mg/mL
   What volume of the re-constituted mixture should be drawn up for injection if the prescription is for
   a. 100 mg   b. 150 mg   c. 200 mg of ampicillin?

4. *The label on vial:* Keflin 1 g
   Re-constitution: Add 4 mL of WFI to yield 0.5 g/2.2 mL
   Calculate the volume of re-constituted mixture to be drawn up for injection if the prescription is for
   a. 200 mg   b. 300 mg   c. 350 mg of Keflin.

5. A girl is to receive amoxicillin 160 mg IV. What volume of solution should be drawn up for injection if the concentration, after dilution with WFI, is
   a. 100 mg/mL   b. 200 mg/mL   c. 250 mg/mL?

6. A vial of ampicillin 500 mg is re-constituted with 1.8 mL of WFI to give a concentration of 250 mg/mL. Calculate the volume of this solution that should be drawn up for injection if the prescription is for
   a. 75 mg   b. 80 mg   c. 175 mg   d. 180 mg.

Check your answers in Chapter 8.

9. DETERMINING A CHILD'S BODY SURFACE AREA USING A NOMOGRAM

As indicated in Section 3, the dosages for the administration of medication to paediatric patients may be based on *BSA*. BSA is a major factor in heat loss and moisture loss from the body. For most medications, the weight of a child is used to calculate the dosage. However, when using certain medications (e.g., cytotoxic medication, which can have severe side effects), BSA gives a more precise measurement than weight.

Fig. 6.3 is a chart called a nomogram that relates a person's height (or length), weight and BSA. Once the height (or length) and weight of a patient have been measured, then the BSA can be determined using the nomogram.

Children of the same age have a wide range of heights (or lengths) and weights and, consequently, a wide range of BSA.

For instance, if a child has a height of 85 cm and a weight of 15 kg, then the child's BSA is found by linking the height and weight measurements with a straight edge (e.g., a ruler): the area is 0.61 m^2.

Additional: An alternative method for calculating BSA involves the use of the Mosteller formula as indicated below:

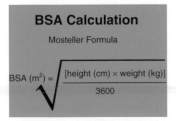

BSA Calculation

Mosteller Formula

$$BSA\ (m^2) = \sqrt{\frac{[height\ (cm) \times weight\ (kg)]}{3600}}$$

Figure 6.2   Mostellar formula for body surface area (BSA) calculation.

This formula, along with examples of others, can appear complex and so awareness of these is useful for alternate methods of calculation. However, these will not be covered in this book.

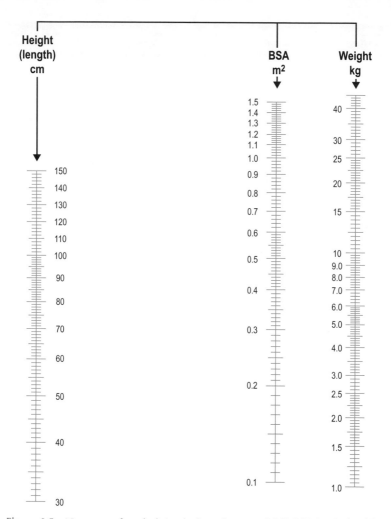

Figure 6.3 Nomogram for calculating body surface area *(BSA)*. BSA is calculated by linking height (or length) and weight with a straight edge (use a ruler).

Example A *Using the nomogram in Fig. 6.3, find the BSA of an infant, aged 6 months, with a length of 65 cm and a weight of 8.2 kg.*

On the nomogram, join length 66 cm and weight 8.2 kg with a straight edge (e.g., ruler). The straight edge then crosses the body surface area scale (marked BSA) at 0.40 m^2.

Example B *Using the nomogram in Fig. 6.3, determine the BSA of a boy of 2 years of age, height 87 cm, weight 13.5 kg.*

On the nomogram, join height 87 cm and weight 13.5 kg with a straight edge. The straight edge then crosses the BSA scale at 0.58 m^2.

✏ **Exercises 6F** *The lengths (heights) and weights used below represent children from 3 months to 3 years of age. Use the nomogram in Fig. 6.3 to find the BSA of each child.*

Estimate answers to the nearest 0.01 m².

1. a. Length 65 cm, weight 6.4 kg
    b. Length 65 cm, weight 8.2 kg

2. a. Length 73 cm, weight 8.8 kg
    b. Length 73 cm, weight 10.5 kg

3. a. Length 85 cm, weight 11.0 kg
    b. Length 85 cm, weight 13.5 kg

4. a. Height 94 cm, weight 12.5 kg
    b. Height 94 cm, weight 15.5 kg

5. a. Weight 5.7 kg, length 57 cm
    b. Weight 5.7 kg, length 63 cm

6. a. Weight 9.4 kg, length 68 cm
    b. Weight 9.4 kg, length 74 cm

7. a. Weight 11.5 kg, length 78 cm
    b. Weight 11.5 kg, length 86 cm

8. a. Weight 14.0 kg, height 87 cm
    b. Weight 14.0 kg, height 97 cm

9. a. Length 67 cm, weight 10.0 kg
    b. Length 78 cm, weight 9.0 kg

10. a. Weight 13.0 kg, height 90 cm
    b. Weight 14.0 kg, height 81 cm

11. a. Length 85 cm, weight 15 kg
    b. Length 50 cm, weight 4.5 kg

12. a. Length 70 cm, weight 9 kg
    b. Length 40 cm, weight 2 kg

Check your answers in Chapter 8.

10. CALCULATING PAEDIATRIC DOSAGES BASED ON BODY SURFACE AREA

Example *A young patient with leukaemia is to be given his weekly injection of doxorubicin. The recommended dosage is 30 mg/m², and the boy's BSA has been determined at 0.48 m². The stock solution contains doxorubicin 10 mg/5 mL. Calculate the volume to be drawn up for injection.*

$$\text{Dose required (mg)} = \text{Body surface area } (\text{m}^2) \times \text{Recommended dosage } (\text{mg/m}^2)$$
$$= 0.48 \text{ m}^2 \times 30 \text{ mg/m}^2$$
$$= 14.40 \text{ mg}$$

$$\text{Volume required} = \frac{\text{Strength required}}{\text{Stock strength}} \times [\text{Volume of stock solution}]$$

$$\text{VR} = \frac{\text{SR}}{\text{SS}} \times \text{VS}$$

$$= \frac{14.4 \text{ mg}}{10 \text{ mg}} \times 5 \text{ mL}$$

$$= \frac{14.4}{10} \times \frac{5}{1} \text{ mL } [\text{Divide the 5 and the 10 by 5}]$$

$$= \frac{14.4}{2} \text{ mL}$$

$$= 7.2 \text{ mL}$$

✏️ **Exercises 6G** *The aim of this exercise is to introduce the method of calculating medication doses based on BSA. These doses are used in complex situations, such as the treatment of children with leukaemia, and are administered under very strict procedures and supervision.*

Calculate the volume required in each case.

1. *Prescribed:* dactinomycin
   Recommended dosage: 1.5 mg/m^2
   Stock strength: 500 micrograms/mL
   BSA: 0.40 m^2

2. *Prescribed:* bleomycin
   Recommended dosage: 10 units/m^2
   Stock strength: 15 units/5 mL
   BSA: 0.54 m^2

3. *Prescribed:* cytarabine
   Recommended dosage: 120 mg/m^2
   Stock strength: 100 mg/5 mL
   BSA: 0.45 m^2

4. *Prescribed:* daunorubicin
   Recommended dosage: 30 mg/m^2
   Stock strength: 20 mg/5 mL
   BSA: 0.52 m^2

5. *Prescribed:* vincristine
   Recommended dosage: 1.5 mg/m^2
   Stock strength: 1 mg/mL
   BSA: 0.64 m^2

6. *Prescribed:* cyclophosphamide
   Recommended dosage: 1000 mg/m^2
   Stock strength: 1 g/50 mL
   BSA: 0.57 m^2

Check your answers in Chapter 8.

7. *Prescribed:* bleomycin
   Recommended dosage: 10 units/m^2
   Stock strength: 15 units/5 mL
   BSA: 0.48 m^2

8. *Prescribed:* doxorubicin
   Recommended dosage: 30 mg/m^2
   Stock strength: 50 mg/25 mL
   BSA: 0.70 m^2

Check your answers in Chapter 8.

11. CASE SCENARIO

James is a 6-year-old with chronic asthma. He was admitted to the assessment unit with an exacerbation of his chronic asthma. On the initial assessment, James is displaying mild symptoms of respiratory rate of 28 breaths/min and a heart rate of 132 beats/min. He has signs of increased work of breathing, however, can talk in sentences.

James is reviewed by the doctor who prescribes him combination therapy of inhaled bronchodilators and oral prednisolone.

1. Calculate the dose for the following medications:
   a. The doctor prescribes salbutamol for mild acute asthma at 10 puffs from a metered dose inhaler every 20 min. Each puff is equivalent to 100 micrograms of salbutamol. How many puffs are prescribed in micrograms for each 20 min?
   b. The prescription for prednisone for children aged between 1 month and 11 years is 2 mg/kg once daily (max dose 60 mg). **James weighs 20 kg.** What is the required dose in milligrams?
   c. Prednisolone is supplied as 5 mg soluble tablets. How many tablets are required?

On review, James' condition is deteriorating and he is displaying signs of moderate acute asthma. The doctor determines that a loading dose of IV magnesium sulphate is required.

2. Calculate the dose for the following medications:
   a. The prescription for IV magnesium sulphate for children with acute asthma aged 2−17 years is 40 mg/kg to be infused over 20 min. What is the dose required in milligrams?
   b. Magnesium sulphate is supplied as 500 mg/1 millilitres solution for injection. What amount of medication in millilitres is the required dose for the infusion?

In addition to magnesium sulphate, James is prescribed oral potassium chloride for the prevention of hypokalaemia.

3. Calculate the dose for the following medications:
   a. The prescription for oral potassium chloride is 2 mmol/kg to be given once daily. What is the required dose for James in mmol? (1 mmol is equal to 18 mg)

b. What is James' dose of oral potassium chloride in milligrams?

c. Potassium chloride oral solution is supplied in ampoules containing 75 mg/1 mL. What is the required dose for James in millilitres?

James is admitted to the ward for assessment and monitoring. You initiate a recorded chart of his fluid balance.

4. Based on the chart below, calculate the totals for fluid intake and output columns and then the fluid balance for James:

Fluid intake			Fluid output	
Time	Oral input amount (mL)		Time	Urine output (mL)
08:00	55		07:00	125
09:00	30		09:40	72
10:30	90		13:15	144
11:30	120			
12:00	55			
13:00	60			
(a) Total input:		(c) Fluid balance:	(b) Total output:	

James is reluctant to drink and so the doctor prescribes IV maintenance fluids containing 0.9% NaCl, 5% glucose and 10 mmol/KCl.

5. Based on James weight calculate his daily maintenance:

a. Note that treatment protocols may vary. For the purpose of this case, the fluid maintenance is to be given in millilitres over a 24-hour period (daily maintenance).

Protocol for daily maintenance:

100 mL/kg up to the first 10 kg of body weight

50 mL/kg for every kg over 10 up to 20 kg of body weight

20 mL/kg for every kg over 20

b. Finally, calculate the hourly infusion rate to be given by a fluid pump. See Chapter 5 for guidance on IV infusion.

7 Case scenario: the life of Maisy

CHAPTER CONTENTS

1. ONE-MONTH-OLD MAISY

One-month-old Maisy was admitted to the assessment unit after her mother reported concerns of reduced feeding. Up until a few days ago, Maisy was feeding well; however, in the last 48 hrs, she has a reduced oral intake.

On initial assessment, the nurse checks Maisy's baby records and notes that her weight last week was 4.5 kg. Today Maisy weighs 4.43 kg.

Questions

1. How much weight has Maisy lost in a week in grams?

   Tip: first convert different weights to grams.

Maisy is bottle fed on formula milk, taking on average 4 ounces (oz) every four hrs. There are 30 mL in every ounce.

2. a. How much milk in millilitres does Maisy take each feed?

   b. Calculate the total expected fluid input for Maisy in millilitres for a 24-hrs period.

The reviewing doctor asks the nurse to keep a record of Maisy's fluid intake over the next 24 hrs. It is recorded by the nurse as follows:

Time	Amount (mL)
07:00	100
11:00	110
14:30	95
18:30	110
23:00	95

3. a. Calculate the total fluid intake for the last 24 hrs.

   b. Based upon your answer from question 2b, calculate the difference between the expected fluid intake and the recorded fluid intake over a 24 hr period.

On initial assessment, the nurse checks with the mother whether Maisy has been having regular wet nappies. A nappy is produced, which the nurse decides to weigh.

The wet nappy containing only urine weighs 260 g. A dry nappy from the same manufacturer weighs 26 g (1 g is equal to 1 mL).

Check your answers in chapter 8.

4. Calculate the amount of urine in millilitres that the initial nappy contained.

Maisy's nappies are weighed for the next 24 hrs and recorded on the fluid output chart:

Time	Amount(mL)
07:00	105
11:00	100
14:30	100
18:30	120
23:00	100

5. a. Calculate the total fluid output for Maisy.
   b. Based on your answer from question 3a, calculate the fluid balance for Maisy.

An ear, nose and throat examination is conducted on initial assessment, and a diagnosis of oral thrush (candida) is made. Oral fluconazole is prescribed.

The prescription for oral fluconazole for an infant aged one month is 3 mg to be given once daily.

Fluconazole oral suspension comes as 50 mg/5 mL.

6. What is the required dose of fluconazole in millilitres to be administered to Maisy?

In addition to fluconazole, paracetamol is prescribed for the pain caused by thrush.

The prescription for paracetamol for an infant aged one month is 30–60 mg every 8 hrs.

Paracetamol oral suspension comes as 120 mg/5 mL.

7. Calculate the required dose for:
   a. 30 mg   b. 60 mg

Check your answers in chapter 8.

2. MAISY AGED 6 YEARS

Six-year-old Maisy is at a children's party for her school friend. Maisy is given some chocolate cake containing a trace of nuts, of which Maisy is allergic. An allergic reaction follows and an ambulance is called.

Maisy arrives to you in the emergency department displaying the following symptoms:

Audible stridor, cyanosis and oxygen saturations of 92% on 15 L of oxygen. Rapid breathing and tachycardia. You can see visible swelling to her face and erythema. Maisy is drowsy and confused. A dose of intramuscular (IM) adrenaline is prescribed by the assessing doctor.

Case scenario: the life of Maisy

Questions

1. The dose of IM adrenaline for a child aged 6–12 years is 300 micrograms of 1:1000 in this case. Adrenaline 1:1000 is supplied as 1 mg/1 mL. What is the required dose in millilitres?

Following the administration of IM adrenaline, intravenous access is gained and a fluid maintenance of 20 mL/kg crystalloid solution is prescribed. Maisy had not been weighed recently and so an estimated weight is required.

2. a. Based on the below formula, calculate the estimated weight in kg for Maisy:

   Weight (in kg) for children aged between 6–12 years = (Age × 3) + 7

   b. Once the estimate weight is obtained, calculate the amount of fluid maintenance required.

Following the commencement of fluid maintenance, a second line of drugs in the form of the steroid hydrocortisone is prescribed.

3. The required dose of IV hydrocortisone for a child aged 6–12 years is 100 mg in this case. Stock strength of hydrocortisone solution for injection is 25 mg/1 mL. Calculate the required dose in millilitres.

Additional options for second-line drugs in the management of anaphylaxis also include Chlorphenamine.

4. The required dose of IV Chlorphenamine for a child aged 6–12 years is 15 mg in this case. Stock strength of Chlorphenamine solution for injection is 10 mg/1 mL. Calculate the required dose in millilitres.

The treatment implemented for the management of anaphylaxis is successful in reducing the severity of symptoms. As a side effect, Maisy is experiencing nausea. Maisy is prescribed IV ondansetron for the nausea symptoms.

5. a. Ondansetron is prescribed at 100 mcg/kg. Calculate the required dose in micrograms.

   b. Convert the required dose from micrograms to milligrams.

   c. Stock strength of ondansetron hydrochloride as solution for injection is 2 mg/1 mL. Calculate the required dose in millilitres.

Check your answers in chapter 8.

3. MAISY AGED 12 YEARS

12-Year-old Maisy is attending the assessment unit experiencing pain and discomfort when she passes urine. She has a high temperature and looks hot and flushed. A urine analysis determines that Maisy has a urinary tract infection.

Questions

1. a. Estimate the weight of Maisy based upon the below calculation:
      Weight (in kg) for children aged between 6—12 years = (Age × 3) + 7
   b. Oral trimethoprim 200 mg every 8 hrs is prescribed. Stock strength is 10 mg/mL. Calculate the required single dose in mL.

Maisy is also prescribed paracetamol for her discomfort. As the nurse, you ask Maisy her preferred method of oral administration. Maisy informs you she is able to take tablets as well as liquid suspension.

Paracetamol 750 mg is prescribed every 4—6 hrs.

2. a. Stock strength of paracetamol liquid suspension is 250 mg/5 mL. Calculate the required dose in millilitres.
   b. Alternatively, paracetamol is available in 500 mg tablets. Calculate the number of tablets required.
   c. The prescription indicated no more than 4 doses in 24 hrs. What is the maximum daily dose not to be exceeded in millilitres?
   d. Convert this from milligrams to grams.

Due to her illness and pyrexia, Maisy has been reluctant to drink. On assessment, she has mild signs of dehydration. Before Maisy is fit for discharge, the assessing doctor asks the nurse to commence rehydration therapy.

Based upon Maisy's weight and fluid requirement in 24 hrs, the doctor encourages the nurse to give 10 mL of clear fluid every 10 min.

3. Calculate the required amount of expected oral intake in 1 hr.

Check your answers in chapter 8.

4. The fluid intake for the next hour is as follows:

Time	Amount (mL)
09:10	8
09:20	10
09:30	8
09:40	8
09:50	10
10:00	10

a. What is the total input for the hour?
b. What is the difference in millilitres compared with the expected amount?

A short time after receiving the oral dose of trimethoprim, Maisy starts to feel nauseous and vomits. The doctor decides to change the prescription of current antibiotic to nitrofurantoin 100 mg every 12 hrs.

5. Stock strength of nitrofurantoin liquid suspension is 25 mg/5 mL. Calculate the required single dose in millilitres.

Check your answers in chapter 8.

4. MAISY AGED 15 YEARS

Maisy is an avid horse rider and unfortunately is attending the emergency department after being kicked by her horse.

Maisy is in the triage room and informs you that her pain is currently 8 out of 10 (10 being the worst pain). She looks pale, tense and is guarding her leg. The nurse as part of a nurse initiated protocol prescribes a one-off dose of paracetamol 750 mg.

Questions

1. Stock strength of paracetamol is 500 mg tablets. Calculate the required dose in tablets.

Maisy is reviewed by the doctor and prescribed morphine for pain. Initially as an IV injection, followed by a continuous IV infusion.

2. Morphine 5 mg is prescribed as an initial IV injection to be given over 5 min. Stock strength is morphine sulphate 10 mg/10 mL. Calculate the required dose in millilitres.

3. Continuous infusion is prescribed as 20 microgram/kg/hr. Maisy weighs 50 kg.
   a. Calculate the required dose for Maisy in micrograms required every hour.
   b. Stock strength is morphine sulphate 10 mg/10 mL. Calculate the required dose in millilitres per hour.

After an hour of commencing IV morphine, Maisy starts to feel nauseous. Following review, the doctor prescribes cyclizine.

4. The dose prescribed is cyclizine 50 mg to be given by IV injection every 8 hrs.

Stock strength of cyclizine solution for injection is 50 mg/mL. Calculate the required dose in millilitres.

5. Cyclizine can be given no more than three times per day. Calculate the maximum daily requirement in milligrams.

Check your answers in chapter 8.

5. MAISY AGED 26 YEARS

Maisy started her nursing career a couple of years ago. She works in the orthopaedic trauma unit. The work is rewarding, however, Maisy finds the shift work tiring. To maintain her health, Maisy takes a combined multivitamin every day containing B_{12}, C, magnesium, calcium and zinc. The recommended daily intake of B_{12} (Cyanocobalamin) for adults is 2.4 microgram. The multivitamin Maisy uses is an effervescent tablet containing 10 microgram of B_{12} per tablet.

Questions

1. Is this stock supplying more or less of the recommended daily intake of B_{12} in each tablet?

2. What is the difference between the stock strength and the recommended daily intake dosage?

Maisy knows that higher doses of vitamin B are safe because the body will only absorb as much as it needs. The same tablet contains 500 mg of vitamin C (ascorbic acid). The recommended daily intake of vitamin C is 65–90 mg, and the upper limit of dosage for vitamin C is 2000 mg/day.

3. If Maisy took enough of these tablets to reach the upper daily limit of vitamin C, how many tablets would she take in one day?

4. If she took that many tablets, how much vitamin B_{12} would she be ingesting?

Maisy has researched this vitamin supplement and understands the limits. She takes only one tablet each day.

Maisy recently injured her wrist during a manual handling incident at work. The doctor prescribed rest, elevation and analgesia.

5. How many 30 mg tablets of codeine should Maisy take if codeine 15 mg is prescribed?

6. If the maximum dose is 60 mg each dose, how many tablets can Maisy take at one time?

Constipation is an adverse effect of taking codeine. Maisy is aware of this and so decides to take a prophylactic laxative. The medicine form is oral liquid.

7. What is the formula for calculating the correct dose?

8. What dose in mg of the active ingredient is ingested in a 15 mL dose if the laxative solution contains 667 g/L?

The maximum daily dose of the laxative solution is 45 mL.

9. How many more mL of the laxative solution can Maisy take in one day to reach the highest dose?

Whilst taking the laxative, it is important to maintain an adequate fluid intake. Two litres per day is recommended. Today, Maisy drank 4 glasses of water each containing 280 mL.

10. How much more fluid does she need to reach the daily requirement?

Check your answers in chapter 8.

6. MAISY AGED 42 YEARS: PRE-OPERATIVE PHASE

Now at age 42, Maisy has a family and a steady career. She has gastroesophageal reflux and takes a daily dose of pantoprazole.

Questions

1. How many 40 mg tablets does she need for a dose of 40 mg?

Today, a sudden bout of cholecystitis has meant that Maisy is hospitalized for a cholecystectomy. In preparation for surgery, the anaesthetist prescribes IV maintenance fluids at 30 mL/kg/day.

2. How many milliliters per day will be infused if Maisy weighs 67 kg?

3. How many mL/h does the infusion pump need to be set at to deliver the full fluid maintenance does in 1 day?

4. What is the formula to determine the volume to be infused when using an infusion pump?

5. Calculate the volume of fluid that will be infused in 12 hrs if the rate is incorrectly set at 1.5 mL/kg/hr.

6. Convert the mL volume from question 5 into litres.

7. Is the daily volume of fluid in question 6 more or less than Maisy's maintenance requirement?

8. What is the formula to calculate the drip rate per minute if the maintenance fluid is delivered by a giving set that delivers 20 drops/mL?

9. Use the formula from the answer to question 8 to calculate the rate if the order for IV fluid is changed to 1 L 8 hrly. Round the result to the nearest whole number.

10. How many millilitres per minute would an infusion pump be set at to deliver the amount of fluid prescribed in question 9?

Check your answers in chapter 8.

7. MAISY AGED 42 YEARS: POST-OPERATIVE PHASE

After the cholecystectomy, Maisy is prescribed patient-controlled analgesia using pethidine 400 mg in 500 mL of normal saline. The solution is to be infused by an infusion pump between 10 and 40 mL/hr, depending on the pain assessment.

Questions

1. Calculate the concentration of the pethidine in saline solution.
2. How many milligrams of pethidine will Maisy receive hourly if the pump is set at 15 mL/hr?
3. At what rate should the pump be set to deliver 20 mg/hr? Give the answer to the nearest whole number.

Check your answers in chapter 8.

8. MAISY AGED 78 YEARS

For the past few years Maisy, has developed several chronic conditions — diabetes, heart disease and idiopathic pulmonary fibrosis.

Maisy takes atenolol for hypertension.

Gatford and Phillips' Drug Calculations

Questions

1. How many 50 mg tablets of atenolol are needed for a dose of atenolol 125 mg?

Maisy takes warfarin as prophylaxis for blood clots. Warfarin tablets are available in strengths of 2 mg, 5 mg and 10 mg. Choose the best combination of whole tablets for the following dosages:

2. a. 8 mg
    b. 12 mg
    c. 16 mg

To relieve the respiratory distress, Maisy is prescribed morphine 45 mg in 500 mL of 0.9% sodium chloride at 10–40 mL/hr. A volumetric infusion pump is to be used to infuse the solution.

3. a. Calculate the concentration (milligrams per millilitre) of the morphine/saline solution.
    b. How many milligrams of morphine will Maisy receive hourly if the pump is set at 25 mL/hr?
    c. At what rate should the pump be set to deliver morphine 3 mg/hr? Give answer to the nearest whole number.

To control the diabetes, Maisy uses combination therapy including insulin. Insulin is supplied in a 10 mL multi-use vial containing 100 units of rapidly acting insulin per millilitres.

4. How many units of insulin are in each vial?
5. How many mL from this vial should you draw up to deliver 22 units of insulin?
6. What type and sized syringe would you use for this dose?

Check your answers in chapter 8.

7. What unit dose of insulin is drawn up in the image below if 0.01 mL is equal to 1 unit?

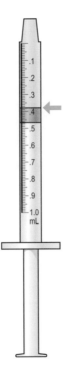

Check your answers in chapter 8.

Maisy is undergoing a chemotherapy regimen to reduce the progression of the idiopathic pulmonary fibrosis. Two hundred milligrams of nintedanib is prescribed twice daily on days 2—21 inclusive of the treatment regimen cycle. Maisy is supplied 100 capsules of 100 mg nintedanib.

8. How many milligrams of the medication will Maisy ingest during one full cycle of her treatment?

Maisy had some adverse effects from the medication and decided to discontinue them after day 15.

9. How many capsules were missed from Maisy's prescribed treatment?

Maisy is taking an oral liquid local anaesthetic to manage the pain of mouth ulcers. Xylocaine viscous 15 mL is prescribed. The stock solution is 20 mg/mL in a 200 mL bottle.

10. How much of the drug in mg is in each dose?

Check your answers in chapter 8.

Answers | 8

DIAGNOSTIC TEST

				Review exercise
1. a. 830	b. 8300	c. 83,000		2A
2. a. 0.258	b. 2.58	c. 25.8		2A
3. a. 0.378	b. 0.0378	c. 0.00378		2B
4. a. 56.9	b. 5.69	c. 0.569		2B
5. a. 1000	b. 1000	c. 1000	d. 1000	2C
6. a. 830 g	b. 6.4 kg			2C
7. a. 780 mg	b. 0.034 g			2C
8. a. 86 micrograms	b. 0.294 mg			2C
9. a. 2400 mL	b. 0.965 L			2C
10. a. 70 mL	b. 7 mL	c. 0.07 L is larger		2D
11. a. 45 mg	b. 450 mg	c. 0.45 g is heavier		2D
12. a. 27	b. 2.7	c. 0.27	d. 0.0027	2E
13. a. 468	b. 4.68	c. 4.68	d. 0.468	2E
14. 2, 3, 4, 6 and 12 are factors				2F
15. 2, 3, 6, 7 and 9 are factors				2F
16. a. $\frac{2}{3}$	b. $\frac{7}{9}$	c. $\frac{1}{15}$ d. $\frac{7}{16}$ e. $\frac{2}{3}$ f. $\frac{2}{5}$		2G
17. a. $\frac{13}{4}$	b. $\frac{11}{2}$	c. $\frac{25}{4}$ d. $\frac{35}{6}$ e. $\frac{16}{5}$ f. $\frac{12}{5}$		2I
18. a. $\frac{2}{3}$	b. $\frac{9}{10}$	c. $\frac{400}{9}$ d. $\frac{9}{5}$ e. $\frac{185}{2}$ f. $\frac{1}{10}$		2J
19. a. 0.7	b. 1.8	c. 0.4		2K
20. a. 0.37	b. 2.63	c. 0.52		2K
21. a. 0.625	b. 0.45	c. 0.68	d. 0.775	2L
22. a. 0.2	b. 0.4	c. 0.8		2M
23. a. 0.71	b. 0.56			2M
24. a. 31.6 $\Rightarrow$ 32	b. 56.2 $\Rightarrow$ 56			2N

Gatford and Phillips' Drug Calculations

			Review exercise
25.	a. 9.16 ⇒ 9.2	b. 7.22 ⇒ 7.2	2N
26.	a. $8\frac{1}{2}$	b. $22\frac{1}{3}$ c. $22\frac{3}{5}$	2O
27.	a. $\frac{11}{4}$	b. $\frac{77}{6}$ c. $\frac{142}{5}$	2O
28.	a. $\frac{5}{9}$	b. $1\frac{1}{14}$ c. $\frac{2}{5}$	2P
29.	a. $\frac{15}{4} = 3\frac{3}{4}$	b. $\frac{5}{2} = 2\frac{1}{2}$	2Q
30.	a. 2.2	b. 1.2	2Q
31.	a. 1030 hrs	b. 2115 hrs	2R
32.	a. 7:30 a.m.	b. 6:50 p.m.	2R
33.	0745 hrs Sunday		2R

Review exercise 2A *Multiplication by 10, 100 and 1000*

1. 6.8, 68, 680
2. 9.75, 97.5, 975
3. 56.2, 562, 5620
4. 770, 7700, 77,000
5. 8250, 82,500, 825,000
6. 2, 20, 200
7. 0.46, 4.6, 46
8. 0.147, 1.47, 14.7
9. 0.06, 0.6, 6
10. 0.75, 7.5, 75
11. 0.8, 8, 80
12. 0.505, 5.05, 50.5

Review exercise 2B *Division by 10, 100 and 1000*

1. 9.84, 0.984, 0.0984
2. 0.591, 0.0591, 0.00591
3. 0.26, 0.026, 0.0026
4. 30.7, 3.07, 0.307
5. 8.2, 0.82, 0.082
6. 0.7, 0.07, 0.007
7. 6.8, 0.68, 0.068
8. 0.229, 0.0229, 0.00229
9. 5.14, 0.514, 0.0514
10. 91.6, 9.16, 0.916
11. 0.894, 0.0894, 0.00894
12. 0.0707, 0.00707, 0.000707

✏ Review exercise 2C *Converting units*

Grams

1. 5000	2. 2400	3. 750	4. 1625

Kilograms

5. 7	6. 0.935	7. 0.085	8. 0.003

Milligrams

9. 4000	11. 690	13. 6	15. 4280
10. 8700	12. 20	14. 655	

Grams

16. 7.25	17. 0.865	18. 0.002

Micrograms

19. 600	21. 75	23. 1
20. 750	22. 80	24. 625

Milligrams

25. 0.825	27. 0.01	29. 0.2
26. 0.065	28. 0.005	

Millilitres

30. 2000	32. 1500	34. 1600	36. 800
31. 30,000	33. 4500	35. 2240	37. 750

Litres

38. 4	40. 0.625	42. 0.005
39. 10	41. 0.095	

Gatford and Phillips' Drug Calculations

✎ **Review exercise 2D** *Comparing measurements*

1. a. 100 mL	b. 10 mL	c. 0.1 L
2. a. 3 mL	b. 300 mL	c. 0.3 L
3. a. 50 mL	b. 5 mL	c. 0.05 L
4. a. 47 mL	b. 470 mL	c. 0.47 L
5. a. 400 mg	b. 4 mg	c. 0.4 g
6. a. 60 mg	b. 600 mg	c. 0.6 g
7. a. 70 mg	b. 7 mg	c. 0.07 g
8. a. 630 mg	b. 63 mg	c. 0.63 g
9. a. 2 micrograms	b. 20 micrograms	c. 0.02 mg
10. a. 900 micrograms	b. 90 micrograms	c. 0.9 mg
11. a. 1 micrograms	b. 100 micrograms	c. 0.1 mg
12. a. 580 micrograms	b. 58 micrograms	c. 0.58 mg
13. a. 1500 g	b. 1050 g	c. 1.5 kg
14. a. 2080 g	b. 2800 g	c. 2.8 kg
15. a. 950 g	b. 95 g	c. 0.95 kg
16. a. 3350 g	b. 3500 g	c. 3.5 kg

✎ **Review exercise 2E** *Multiplication of decimals*

1. 45, 4.5, 0.45, 0.45
2. 14, 0.14, 0.014, 0.0014
3. 12, 0.12, 0.12, 0.0012
4. 56, 5.6, 0.56, 0.0056
5. 102, 10.2, 1.02, 0.102
6. 152, 15.2, 0.152, 0.152
7. 145, 1.45, 1.45, 1.45
8. 93, 0.93, 0.0093, 0.093
9. 333, 33.3, 0.333, 0.0333
10. 287, 0.287, 0.0287, 2.87
11. 616, 6.16, 0.0616, 0.616
12. 768, 0.768, 0.0768, 0.0768

Review exercise 2F *Factors*

1. 2, 4, 5
2. 3, 4, 12
3. 3, 5, 15
4. 2, 8, 14
5. 3, 4, 12, 15, 20
6. 3, 4, 6, 12, 18
7. 3, 5, 15, 25
8. 5, 17
9. 3, 8, 12, 16, 24
10. 5, 20, 25
11. 4, 9, 12, 18
12. 3, 5, 12, 15
13. 3, 5, 9, 15
14. 4, 8, 12, 16, 18, 24
15. 5, 15, 25

Review exercise 2G *Simplifying fractions I*

Part i

1. 4
2. $\dfrac{5}{7}$
3. $\dfrac{3}{8}$
4. $\dfrac{1}{2}$

5. $\dfrac{5}{7}$
6. $\dfrac{5}{6}$
7. $\dfrac{4}{5}$
8. $\dfrac{3}{7}$

9. $\dfrac{7}{8}$
10. $\dfrac{2}{3}$
11. $\dfrac{8}{9}$
12. $\dfrac{1}{3}$

13. $\dfrac{9}{14}$
14. $\dfrac{13}{16}$
15. $\dfrac{3}{10}$

Part ii

1. $\dfrac{1}{2}$
2. $\dfrac{3}{8}$
3. $\dfrac{3}{10}$
4. $\dfrac{1}{2}$

5. $\dfrac{5}{12}$
6. $\dfrac{5}{16}$
7. $\dfrac{2}{15}$
8. $\dfrac{8}{35}$

9. $\dfrac{4}{25}$
10. $\dfrac{3}{4}$
11. $\dfrac{11}{16}$
12. $\dfrac{4}{9}$

13. $\dfrac{7}{9}$
14. $\dfrac{3}{4}$
15. $\dfrac{17}{24}$
16. $\dfrac{13}{30}$

Review exercise 2H *Simplifying fractions II*

1. $\dfrac{3}{5}$

2. $\dfrac{2}{3}$

3. $\dfrac{5}{12}$

4. $\dfrac{5}{6}$

5. $\dfrac{13}{15}$

6. $\dfrac{2}{5}$

7. $\dfrac{3}{4}$

8. $\dfrac{3}{8}$

9. $\dfrac{2}{3}$

10. $\dfrac{9}{10}$

11. $\dfrac{9}{10}$

12. $\dfrac{6}{25}$

13. $\dfrac{14}{25}$

14. $\dfrac{7}{10}$

15. $\dfrac{5}{6}$

16. $\dfrac{1}{6}$

17. $\dfrac{3}{10}$

18. $\dfrac{11}{16}$

✏ **Review exercise 2I** *Simplifying fractions III*

1. a. $\dfrac{3}{2}$ b. $\dfrac{5}{2}$ c. $\dfrac{15}{4}$ d. $\dfrac{17}{4}$

2. a. $\dfrac{25}{2}$ b. $\dfrac{75}{4}$ c. $\dfrac{75}{2}$ d. $\dfrac{375}{4}$

3. a. $\dfrac{25}{2}$ b. $\dfrac{175}{6}$ c. $\dfrac{125}{3}$ d. $\dfrac{250}{3}$

4. a. $\dfrac{5}{2}$ b. $\dfrac{15}{2}$ c. $\dfrac{19}{2}$ d. $\dfrac{55}{4}$

5. a. $\dfrac{7}{5}$ b. $\dfrac{3}{2}$ c. $\dfrac{12}{5}$ d. $\dfrac{5}{2}$

6. a. $\dfrac{4}{3}$ b. $\dfrac{5}{2}$ c. $\dfrac{25}{2}$ d. $\dfrac{50}{3}$

7. a. $\dfrac{5}{4}$ b. $\dfrac{5}{2}$ c. $\dfrac{55}{8}$ d. $\dfrac{25}{2}$

8. a. $\dfrac{3}{2}$ b. $\dfrac{5}{3}$ c. $\dfrac{5}{2}$ d. $\dfrac{15}{4}$

9. a. $\dfrac{8}{5}$ b. $\dfrac{12}{5}$ c. $\dfrac{32}{5}$ d. $\dfrac{36}{5}$

10. a. $\dfrac{6}{5}$ b. $\dfrac{14}{5}$ c. $\dfrac{22}{5}$ d. $\dfrac{38}{5}$

11. a. $\dfrac{6}{5}$ b. $\dfrac{3}{2}$ c. $\dfrac{8}{3}$ d. $\dfrac{19}{3}$

12. a. $\dfrac{16}{5}$ b. $\dfrac{18}{5}$ c. $\dfrac{24}{5}$ d. $\dfrac{36}{5}$

Gatford and Phillips' Drug Calculations

✎ Review exercise 2J *Simplifying fractions IV*

1. $\dfrac{4}{5}$	5. 2	9. $\dfrac{5}{2}$	13. 200
2. $\dfrac{3}{4}$	6. $\dfrac{7}{10}$	10. $\dfrac{19}{8}$	14. $\dfrac{200}{9}$
3. $\dfrac{3}{2}$	7. $\dfrac{9}{4}$	11. 80	15. $\dfrac{1000}{11}$
4. $\dfrac{3}{7}$	8. $\dfrac{11}{2}$	12. $\dfrac{200}{3}$	16. $\dfrac{9}{2}$

✎ Review exercise 2K *Rounding off decimal numbers*

Part i

1. 0.9	4. 0.6	7. 2.4	10. 1.1
2. 0.5	5. 1.0	8. 1.1	11. 3.0
3. 0.9	6. 1.6	9. 0.2	12. 1.0

Part ii

1. 0.33	4. 0.14	7. 2.71	10. 0.63
2. 1.67	5. 0.13	8. 1.29	11. 0.78
3. 0.88	6. 0.92	9. 0.64	12. 2.43

✎ Review exercise 2L *Fraction to a decimal I*

1. 0.5	6. 0.875	11. 0.04	16. 0.675
2. 0.25	7. 0.05	12. 0.32	17. 0.14
3. 0.75	8. 0.35	13. 0.88	18. 0.86
4. 0.2	9. 0.65	14. 0.025	
5. 0.6	10. 0.95	15. 0.225	

Answers

Review exercise 2M *Fraction to a decimal II*

Part i

1. 0.3
2. 0.8
3. 0.7
4. 0.2
5. 0.5
6. 0.9

Part ii

1. 0.67
2. 0.17
3. 0.86
4. 0.89
5. 0.36
6. 0.42

Review exercise 2N *Fraction to a decimal III*

Part i

1. 33.3 ⇒ 33
2. 83.3 ⇒ 83
3. 166.6 ⇒ 167
4. 31.2 ⇒ 31
5. 14.4 ⇒ 14
6. 28.8 ⇒ 29
7. 45.8 ⇒ 46
8. 34.2 ⇒ 34
9. 42.8 ⇒ 43
10. 46.8 ⇒ 47
11. 53.1 ⇒ 53
12. 61.1 ⇒ 61

Part ii

1. 1.66 ⇒ 1.7
2. 3.33 ⇒ 3.3
3. 5.83 → 5.8
4. 4.16 ⇒ 4.2
5. 2.85 ⇒ 2.9
6. 3.57 ⇒ 3.6
7. 7.14 ⇒ 7.1
8. 9.28 ⇒ 9.3
9. 6.87 ⇒ 6.9
10. 5.62 ⇒ 5.6
11. 7.77 ⇒ 7.8
12. 9.44 ⇒ 9.4

✎ Review exercise 2O *Mixed numbers and improper fractions*

Part i

1. $2\frac{1}{2}$ 4. $5\frac{1}{7}$ 7. $17\frac{3}{4}$ 10. $14\frac{3}{7}$

2. $3\frac{2}{3}$ 5. $5\frac{4}{9}$ 8. $17\frac{1}{5}$ 11. $14\frac{1}{8}$

3. $4\frac{2}{5}$ 6. $21\frac{2}{3}$ 9. $15\frac{5}{6}$ 12. $13\frac{8}{9}$

Part ii

1. $\frac{3}{2}$ 4. $\frac{14}{3}$ 7. $\frac{67}{6}$ 10. $\frac{45}{2}$

2. $\frac{4}{3}$ 5. $\frac{25}{4}$ 8. $\frac{133}{8}$ 11. $\frac{111}{4}$

3. $\frac{13}{5}$ 6. $\frac{49}{5}$ 9. $\frac{155}{9}$ 12. $\frac{228}{7}$

✎ Review exercise 2P *Multiplication of fractions*

1. $\frac{1}{5}$ 4. $\frac{3}{5}$ 7. $\frac{11}{42}$ 10. $\frac{9}{10}$

2. $\frac{5}{9}$ 5. $\frac{5}{6}$ 8. $\frac{20}{21}$ 11. $\frac{7}{18}$

3. $1\frac{2}{3}$ 6. $\frac{4}{9}$ 9. $\frac{5}{28}$ 12. $\frac{7}{15}$

✏ **Review exercise 2Q** *Multiplication of a fraction by a whole number*

Part i

1. $\dfrac{15}{4} = 3\dfrac{3}{4}$ 4. $\dfrac{20}{3} = 6\dfrac{2}{3}$ 7. $\dfrac{9}{2} = 4\dfrac{1}{2}$ 10. $\dfrac{10}{3} = 3\dfrac{1}{3}$

2. $\dfrac{6}{5} = 1\dfrac{1}{5}$ 5. 6 8. $\dfrac{15}{8} = 1\dfrac{7}{8}$ 11. $\dfrac{10}{3} = 3\dfrac{1}{3}$

3. 4 6. $\dfrac{6}{7}$ 9. 4 12. $\dfrac{3}{5}$

Part ii

1. 3.5   4. 0.7   7. 3.6   10. 2.8
2. 1.2   5. 2.5   8. 3.75   11. 9
3. 0.6   6. 1.8   9. 1.6   12. 4.4

✏ **Review exercise 2R** *24-hrs time*

Part i

All answers are in hours.

1. 0910   4. 1105   7. 1255   10. 1735
2. 2040   5. 0400   8. 1315   11. 0745
3. 0230   6. 1525   9. 0620   12. 2250

Part ii

1. 7:35 p.m.   4. 2:00 a.m.   7. 9:25 p.m.   10. 5:10 a.m.
2. 10:30 p.m.   5. 1:05 p.m.   8. 6:40 a.m.   11. 12:20 p.m.
3. 1:05 a.m.   6. 5:45 p.m.   9. 11:15 p.m.   12. 2:50 p.m.

Part iii

All answers are in hours.

1. 1745 Monday   5. 0525 Monday
2. 0530 Friday   6. 1840 Wednesday
3. 2015 Saturday   7. 0020 Saturday
4. 0400 Wednesday   8. 1910 Thursday

CHAPTER 3: DOSAGES CALCULATIONS FOR SOLID MEDICATIONS

Exercise 3A

1. 2

2. $\frac{1}{2}$

3. $1\frac{1}{2}$

4. 2

5. $1\frac{1}{2}$

6. $\frac{1}{2}$

7. $1\frac{1}{2}$

8. $\frac{1}{2}$

9. $2\frac{1}{2}$

10. $\frac{1}{2}$

11. 0.6 mg

12. 8

13. 2

14. $\frac{1}{2}$

15. $1\frac{1}{2}$

Exercise 3B

1. a. 2 mg + 2 mg (2 tablets)
   b. 5 mg + 2 mg + 2 mg (3 tablets)
   c. 10 mg + 2 mg (2 tablets)
   d. 10 mg + 5 mg (2 tablets)

2. a. 5 mg + 2 mg (2 tablets)
   b. 5 mg + 2 mg + 2 mg (3 tablets)
   c. 10 mg + 5 mg (2 tablets)
   d. 10 mg + 10 mg (2 tablets)

3. a. 120 mg + 80 mg (2 tablets); or 160 mg + 40 mg (2 tablets)
   b. 120 mg + 120 mg (2 tablets); or 160 mg + 80 mg (2 tablets)
   c. 160 mg + 120 mg (2 tablets)
   d. 160 mg + 160 mg (2 tablets)

4. a. 5 mg + 1 mg (2 tablets)
   b. 5 mg + 2 mg + 1 mg (3 tablets)
   c. 5 mg + 2 mg + 2 mg (3 tablets)
   d. 5 mg + 5 mg + 1 mg (3 tablets)

5. a. 40 mg + 20 mg (2 tablets)
   b. 80 mg + 20 mg (2 tablets)
   c. 80 mg + 80 mg + 40 mg (3 tablets)
   d. 500 mg + 40 mg + 20 mg (3 tablets)

6. a. 25 mg + 10 mg (2 tablets)
   b. 50 mg + 10 mg (2 tablets)
   c. 50 mg + 25 mg (2 tablets)
   d. 100 mg + 10 mg + 10 mg (3 tablets)

7. a. 2 mg + 1 mg (2 tablets)
   b. 5 mg + 2 mg (2 tablets)
   c. 10 mg + 2 mg + 1 mg (3 tablets)
   d. 10 mg + 5 mg + 1 mg (3 tablets)

8. a. 10 mg + 5 mg (2 tablets)
   b. 10 mg + 10 mg (2 tablets)
   c. 10 mg + 10 mg + 5 mg + 1 mg (4 tablets)
   d. 10 mg + 10 mg + 10 mg + 5 mg (4 tablets)

9. a. 50 mg (1 tablet)
   b. 50 mg + 25 mg (2 tablets)
   c. 50 mg + 50 mg + 25 mg (3 tablets)
   d. 50 mg + 50 mg + 50 mg (3 tablets)

10. a. 250 mg (1 tablet)
    b. 100 mg + 100 mg + 100 mg + 100 mg (4 tablets)
    c. 250 mg + 250 mg + 100 mg (3 tablets)
    d. 500 mg + 250 mg (2 tablets)

11. a. 50 mg + 25 mg (2 tablets)
    b. 50 mg + 50 mg (2 tablets)
    c. 50 mg + 50 mg + 25 mg (3 tablets)
    d. 50 mg + 50 mg + 50 mg + 50 mg (4 tablets)

12. a. 40 mg + 20 mg (2 tablets)
    b. 40 mg + 40 mg tablet (2 tablets)
    c. 40 mg + 40 mg + 20 mg (3 tablets)
    d. 40 mg + 40 mg + 40 mg (3 tablets)

Exercise 3E

1. 2 tablets
2. 2 tablets

CASE SCENARIO

1. 5 mg × 2 tablets = 10 mg
2. 5 mg × 3 tablets = 15 mg
3. 2 × 50 mg tablets = 100 mg
4. $\frac{1}{2}$ × 5 mg tablet = 2.5 mg
5. 1 × 50 mg tablet (because the dose is 100 mg divided into two doses).
6. Once, because it is a full dose in a sustained release form.
7. Dose was 15 mg 4th hrly. Therefore, six doses in 24 hrs. Thus, 6 × 15 mg per dose = 90 mg in 24 hrs. Table 1 from NHS identified 37 micrograms patch of fentanyl. However, the protocol suggests commencing at 50% of the oral dose. Therefore, the 12.5 patch should be selected as it is closer to 50% of the 37 micrograms dose than the 25 micrograms patch. Titration to Greg's pain in the future may require an adjustment of the patch dose.
8. 4 wafers
9. 2 tablets
10. 6.30 p.m.

CHAPTER 4: DOSAGES CALCULATIONS FOR LIQUID MEDICATIONS

Exercise 4A *All answers are in milligrams (mg).*

1. a. 20	b. 30	c. 50
2. a. 6	b. 10	c. 14
3. a. 80	b. 200	c. 400
4. a. 500	b. 750	c. 1000
5. a. 40	b. 100	c. 160
6. a. 500	b. 1000	c. 1500
7. a. 50	b. 150	c. 250
8. a. 750	b. 1250	c. 1750
9. a. 50	b. 100	c. 250
10. a. 750	b. 1250	c. 1750

Exercise 4B

1. less than 1 mL	5. equal to 10 mL
2. more than 2 mL	6. less than 2 mL
3. less than 5 mL	7. more than 1 mL
4. more than 2 mL	

Exercise 4C *All answers are in millilitres (mL). Volumes more than 1 mL are given to one decimal place; volumes less than 1 mL are given to two decimal places.*

1. 0.8	3. 0.9	5. 1.5
2. 1.4	4. 1.7	6. 3

Exercise 4D *All answers are in millilitres (mL). Volumes more than 1 mL are given to one decimal place; volumes less than 1 mL are given to two decimal places.*

1. 5	6. 0.2	11. 1.3	16. 4
2. 3.2	7. 1.3	12. 1.2	17. 1.5
3. 0.5	8. 1.6	13. 1.5	18. 0.6
4. 4	9. 0.55	14. 2.5	19. 0.6
5. 0.8	10. 2.5	15. 1.6	20. 3.75 ⇒ 3.8

Exercise 4E *All answers are in millilitres (mL).*

1. 6.7	4. 0.67	7. 1.4
2. 1.3	5. 0.88	8. 1.8
3. 0.83	6. 0.43	9. 1.3

Exercise 4F *All answers are in millilitres (mL).*

1. 0.8	6. 1.6	11. 4	16. 3.8
2. 0.28	7. 1.2	12. 2.4	17. 1.3
3. 12.5	8. 0.8	13. 1.8	18. 0.75
4. 0.6	9. 3	14. 3.8	19. 6
5. 0.35	10. 2.5	15. 0.75	20. 1.3

Exercise 4G *All volumes are in millilitres (mL).*

1. 20	6. 25	11. 15
2. 4	7. 7.5	12. 25
3. 2.5	8. 20	13. 16
4. 7.5	9. 7	14. 15
5. 6	10. 24	15. 2.5

Exercise 4H

1. a. (i) 10 mg (ii) 20 mg
   b. 4 mL
2. a. (i) 25 mg (ii) 50 mg
   b. 8 mL

Exercise 4I *All answers are in millilitres (mL).*

1. 0.8	3. 0.5
2. 6	4. 3.5

Gatford and Phillips' Drug Calculations

Exercise 4J

1. a. $\frac{1}{100}$ mL = 0.01 mL b. A 0.2 mL B 0.38 mL C 0.73 mL D 0.55 mL

2. a. $\frac{1}{10}$ mL = 0.1 mL b. A 1.2 mL B 2.15 mL C 2.6 mL

3. a. $\frac{1}{5}$ mL = 0.2 mL b. A 2.2 mL B 4.5 mL C 3.9 mL

4. a. $\frac{1}{5}$ mL = 0.2 mL b. A 6 mL B 3.4 mL C 7.5 mL

5. a. 2 units b. A 40 units B 4 units C 75 units D 65 units

6. a. 1 unit b. A 30 units B 42 units C 25 units D 17 units

7. a. $\frac{1}{2}$ unit = 0.5 unit b. A 40 units B 36 units C 27.5 units D 32.5 units

CASE SCENARIO

1. 0.84 g × 48 kg = 40.32 g daily
2. 40.32 g divided by 18 g of protein per bottle of energy drink = 2.24 bottles
3. 2.24 bottles of energy drink × 125 mL per bottle = 280 mL of energy drink
4. 280 mL required − 187.5 mL consumed = 92.5 mL
5. 2 mL × 60 min × 24 hrs = 2880 mL
6. 2880 divided by 1000 = 2.88L
7. 0.25 mL
8. 1 mL syringe
9. 4 mL
10. 2 ampoules
11. 0.25 mL
12. 1 mL

CHAPTER 5: DOSAGE CALCULATIONS FOR INFUSED MEDICATIONS

Exercise 5A

1. a. 84 mL   b. 336 mL   c. 504 mL

2. a. 375 mL   b. 625 mL   c. 1500 mL

3. a. 90 mL   b. 150 mL   c. 720 mL

4. 20 hrs

5. $12\frac{1}{2}$ hrs $= 12$ hrs 30 min

6. $6\frac{2}{3}$ hrs $= 6$ hrs 40 min

7. $\frac{2}{3}$ hr $= 40$ min

8. a. 110 mL   b. 275 mL   c. 605 mL

9. $2\frac{1}{2}$ hrs

10. a. 372 mL   b. 744 mL   c. 1488 mL

11. 4 hrs

12. a. 336 mL   b. 840 mL   c. 1176 mL

Exercise 5B *All answers are in mL/hr.*

1. 125
2. 41.6 ⇒ 42
3. 71.4 ⇒ 71
4. 133.3 ⇒ 133
5. 166.6 ⇒ 167
6. 62.5 ⇒ 63
7. 62.5 ⇒ 63
8. 41.6 ⇒ 42
9. 55.5 ⇒ 56
10. 83.3 ⇒ 83
11. 75
12. 90.9 ⇒ 91

Exercise 5C *All answers are in mL/h.*

1. 120	6. 106.6 ⇒ 107
2. 144	7. 112.5 ⇒ 113
3. 200	8. 168
4. 100	9. 160
5. 102.8 ⇒ 103	10. 200

Exercise 5D *All answers are in drops/min.*

1. 50	7. 50
2. 25	8. 120
3. 20.8 ⇒ 21	9. 40
4. 13.8 ⇒ 14	10. 24
5. 27.7 ⇒ 28	11. 80
6. 33.3 ⇒ 33	12. 22.2 ⇒ 22

Exercise 5E *All answers are in drops/min.*

1. 20.8 ⇒ 21	6. 40
2. 41.6 ⇒ 42	7. 34.2 ⇒ 34
3. 41.6 ⇒ 42	8. 35
4. 50	9. 87.5 ⇒ 88
5. 29.1 ⇒ 29	10. 27.7 ⇒ 28

Exercise 5F *All answers are in hours.*

1. 1530 Tuesday	5. 2400 Monday (or 0000 Tuesday)
2. 0100 Monday	
3. 2130 Friday	6. 0600 Sunday
4. 0345 Friday	7. 0030 Thursday

Exercise 5G

1. 1800 mL or 1.8 L
2. Running time = $13\frac{1}{3}$ hrs = 13 hrs 20 min
   Finishing time = 0800 hrs + 13 hrs 20 min = 2120 hrs
3. Running time = 20 hrs
   Finishing time = 2100 hrs Monday +20 hrs 00 min = 1700 hrs Tuesday
4. 6 hrs + 7 hrs = 13 hrs
5. Total running time = 5 hrs + $2\frac{1}{2}$ hrs = $7\frac{1}{2}$ hrs = 7 hrs 30 min
   Finishing time = 0800 hrs + 7 hrs 30 min = 1530 hrs
6. Total running time = 10 hrs + 8 hrs = 18 hrs
   Finishing time = 0430 hrs + 18 hrs 00 min = 2230 hrs
7. 110 mL/hr
8. 55 mL/hr
9. 1620 mL or 1.62 L
10. Running time = 12 hrs 30 min
    Finishing time = 0700 hrs + 12 hrs 30 min = 1930 hrs
11. 6 hrs + 11 hrs = 17 hrs
    Total running time = 8 hrs + 11 hrs = 19 hrs
12. Finishing time = 0300 hrs + 19 hrs 00 min = 2200 hrs

Exercise 5H

1. a. 0.7 mg/mL
   b. i. 7 mg   ii. 10.5 mg   iii. 17.5 mg   iv. 28 mg

   c. i. 12.8 ⇒ 13 mL/hr   ii. 17.1 ⇒ 17 mL/hr
      iii. 28.5 ⇒ 29 mL/hr   iv. 35.7 ⇒ 36 mL/hr

2. a. 0.1 mg/mL
   b. i. 1 mg   ii. 1.5 mg   iii. 2 mg   iv. 4 mg

   c. i. 15 mL/hr   ii. 25 mL/hr   iii. 30 mL/hr   iv. 35 mL/hr

3. a. 10 micrograms/mL   b. 10 micrograms   c. 60 micrograms

4. a. 0.5 mg/mL   b. 2.5 mg/hr   c. 7 mL/hr

5. a. 10 micrograms/mL   b. 10 micrograms   c. 50 micrograms

Exercise 5I

All answers are in kilojoules.

1. 800
2. 2000
3. 1600
4. 2000

5. 0 (no carbohydrate)
6. 480
7. 0 (no carbohydrate)
8. 400

CASE SCENARIO

1. $0.35 \times 79 \times 24 = 663.6$ micrograms
2. $0.35 \times 79 \times 1 = 27.65$ micrograms
3. $663.6/100 \times 2 = 13.272$ mL
4. $663.6/500 \times 10 = 13.272$ mL
5. Stock solution number 2 because there are fewer ampoules to open. Thus, reducing the risk of injury and the cost of resources.
6. 13.272 mL
7. $27.65/663.6 \times 100/1 = 4.16$ mL/hr
8. Cease infusion, monitor vital signs including oxygen saturation, administer oxygen if needed, withhold additional sedation, notify treating team.
9. $60/5 = 12$
10. 12×20 micrograms $= 240$ micrograms
11. 41.6 drops/min rounded to 42 drops/min
12. Due to the risk of overdose and cardiac dysrhythmia

CHAPTER 6: PAEDIATRIC DOSAGES

Exercise 6A *All answers are in milligrams (mg).*

1. 28	4. 120	7. 250	10. 900
2. 99	5. 150	8. 200	11. 240
3. 675	6. 90	9. 225	12. 540

Exercise 6B

1. less than 1 mL	5. more than 1 mL	9. more than 10 mL
2. less than 5 mL	6. less than 3 mL	10. equal to 1 mL
3. more than 2 mL	7. less than 1.5 mL	11. less than 100 mL
4. equal to 1 mL	8. less than 10 mL	12. less than 10 mL

Exercise 6C *All answers are in millilitres (mL). Volumes more than 1 mL are given to one decimal place; volumes less than 1 mL are given to two decimal places.*

1. 0.80	5. 0.48	9. 0.25	13. 1.0
2. 0.75	6. 1.2	10. 7.2	14. 0.80
3. 0.50	7. 1.2	11. 0.65	15. 0.45
4. 0.72	8. 0.30	12. 1.5	16. 0.80

Exercise 6D *All answers are in millilitres (mL). Volumes more than 1 mL are given to one decimal place; volumes less than 1 mL are given to two decimal places.*

1. 3.5	5. 2.5	9. 11.25 $\Rightarrow$ 11.3	13. 4.0
2. 12.5	6. 4.0	10. 2.25 $\Rightarrow$ 2.3	14. 6.0
3. 12.5	7. 8.0	11. 0.60	15. 10
4. 7.0	8. 14.0	12. 0.50	16. 15

Exercise 6E *All answers are in millilitres (mL).*

1. a. 1.2	b. 0.90	c. 0.60	
2. a. 1.5	b. 1.2	c. 0.75	d. 0.60
3. a. 0.40	b. 0.60	c. 0.80	
4. a. 0.88	b. 1.32 $\Rightarrow$ 1.3	c. 1.54 $\Rightarrow$ 1.5	
5. a. 1.6	b. 0.80	c. 0.64	
6. a. 0.30	b. 0.32	c. 0.70	d. 0.72

Exercise 6F *All answers give body surface area (BSA) in m².*

1. a. 0.35 b. 0.40	5. a. 0.31 b. 0.32	9. a. 0.45 b. 0.45
2. a. 0.43 b. 0.48	6. a. 0.43 b. 0.45	10. a. 0.57 b. 0.57
3. a. 0.51 b. 0.57	7. a. 0.51 b. 0.53	11. a. 0.60 b. 0.26
4. a. 0.57 b. 0.64	8. a. 0.59 b. 0.61	12. a. 0.43 b. 0.16

Exercise 6G *All answers are in millilitres (mL).*

1. 1.2	3. 2.7	5. 0.96	7. 1.6
2. 1.8	4. 3.9	6. 28.5	8. 10.5

CASE SCENARIO

1. a. 1000 micrograms   b. 40 mg   c. 8 tablets
2. a. 800 mg   b. 1.6 mL
3. a. 40 mmol   b. 720 mg   c. 9.6 mL
4. a. Total input: 410 mL   b. Total output: 341 mL
   c. Fluid balance: positive '+' 69 mL.
5. a. 1500 mL   b. 62.5 mL/hr

CHAPTER 7: CASE SCENARIO: THE LIFE OF MAISY

1. ONE-MONTH-OLD MAISY

1. 70 g
2. a. 120 mL
   b. 720 mL in 24 hrs (Maisy is fed every 4 hrs, or six times in 24 hrs. Therefore, 120 mL × 6 times per day).
3. a. 510 mL   b. 720 mL − 510 mL = 210 mL
4. 234 mL
5. a. 525 mL
   b. Negative balance of 15 mL (510 mL input minus 525 mL fluid output)
6. 0.3 mL
7. a. 1.25 mL   b. 2.5 mL

2. MAISY AGED 6 YEARS

1. 0.3 mL
2. a. 25 kg   b. 20 mL × 25 kg = 500 mL
3. 4 mL
4. 1 mL
5. a. 100 × 25 = 2500 micrograms   b. 2.5 mg   c. 1.25 mL

3. MAISY AGED 12 YEARS

1. a. 43 kg   b. 20 mL
2. a. 15 mL   b. 1.5 tablets   c. 3000 mg   d. 3 g
3. 60 mL
4. a. 54 mL   b. 6 mL
5. 20 mL

Gatford and Phillips' Drug Calculations

4. MAISY AGED 15 YEARS

1. 1.5 tablets
2. 5 mL
3. a. 1000 micrograms/hr   b. 1 mL
4. 1 mL
5. 150 mg

5. MAISY AGED 26 YEARS

1. More
2. 7.6 micrograms
3. 4 tablets
4. 40 micrograms
5. $\frac{1}{2}$ tablet
6. 2 tablets
7. Volume required $= \frac{\text{Strength required}}{\text{Stock strength}} \times$ [Volumne of stock solution]
8. 10.005 mg
9. 30 mL
10. 880 mL

6. MAISY AGED 42 YEARS: PRE-OPERATIVE PHASE

1. 1 tablet
2. 2010 mL
3. 83.75 mL/hr
4. Volume (mL) = Rate (mL/hr)×Time (hrs)
5. 1206 mL
6. 1.206 L
7. More
8. Rate(drops/min) $= \frac{\text{Volume (mL)} \times \text{Drop factor (drop/mL)}}{\text{Time (min)}}$
9. 41.6 DPM rounded to 42 DPM
10. 125 mL/hr

7. MAISY AGED 42 YEARS: POST-OPERATIVE PHASE

1. 0.8 mg/mL
2. 12 mg/hr
3. 25 mL/hr

8. MAISY AGED 78 YEARS

1. $2\frac{1}{2}$ tablets
2. a. 2 mg + 2 mg + 2 mg + 2 mg (4 tablets)
   b. 10 mg + 2 mg (2 tablets)
   c. 10 mg + 2 mg + 2 mg + 2 mg (4 tablets)
3. a. 0.09 mg/mL
   b. 2.25 mg/hr
   c. 33.3 $\Rightarrow$ 33 mL/hr
4. 1000 units
5. 0.22 mL
6. A 50 unit syringe that is 0.5 mL
7. 38 units
8. 8000 mg (20 day cycle, 2 × 200 mg tablets × 20 days)
9. 12 capsules
10. 300 mg

Index

Note: Page numbers followed by "f" indicate figures, "t" indicate tables and "b" indicate boxes.

Index